contributions to
ASIAN
STUDIES

18

E.J. Brill - Leiden

CONTRIBUTIONS
TO
ASIAN STUDIES

CONTRIBUTIONS TO ASIAN STUDIES

Editors: K. Ishwaran and Bardwell L. Smith

TM.

VOLUME 18

SOUTH ASIAN SYSTEMS OF HEALING

Edited by E. Valentine Daniel and Judy F. Pugh

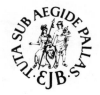

LEIDEN

E. J. BRILL

1984

ISBN   90 04 07085 0

Contents

CONTRIBUTIONS TO ASIAN STUDIES SERIES

Despite socio-cultural, economic, political and geographical diversity, the countries of Asia display certain broad similarities. In general, all of them are products of ancient civilizations, faced with the complex forces of modernity, which they have responded to in quite complex ways. Asia's unity in diversity, the dynamics of its social and cultural patterns, past and present, have stimulated a large body of scholarly work. A new phase in Asian studies has developed through first rate contributions from indigenous scholars who often bring an outlook and understanding of their own. *Contributions to Asian Studies*, a semi-annual publication, is intended as a forum for scholarly analyses of Asian societies and cultures, past and contemporary, from the diverse standpoints of the international community of scholars in all the social sciences and humanities.

Introduction*

E. VALENTINE DANIEL and JUDY F. PUGH

University of Washington, Seattle, U.S.A.
University of British Columbia, Vancouver, Canada

THIS VOLUME OPENS WITH AN ESSAY, written by one who is not a South Asianist, on a subject that is not, prima-facie, South Asian. Rather, it concerns an epistemological problem endemic to medical anthropology, a problem which finds its source in a Cartesian, if not Zwinglian (Oberoi 1978), dualism which makes into God's truth such dichotomies as body and mind, fact and value, theory and practice, symbolic and real, and now, illness and disease. Robert Hahn critically evaluates the medical anthropological literature which has either nurtured and promoted this hocus pocus or has tried but failed to divest itself of it. Following a perspicacious review of the disease-illness dichotomy in the literature and an exposé of the contradictions inherent in it, Hahn suggests, what to a Buddhist may seem only obvious, that for any system of thought concerned with healing, the starting point ought to be the experience of suffering.

The remaining essays in this volume, playing ethnographic Śakti to Hahn's theoretical Puruṣa, have blown life into the body of his analytic argument, and in so doing helped freshen up the intellectual conditions that have remained far too conjested with Cartesian ideas where every second scholar in this crowded environment has been an unwitting carrier of a variant of these conceptual debilitators.

Egnor's gripping essay on the smallpox goddess' role and place in the life of her devotee, Sarasvati, is a study in the texture of suffering. Tuberculosis, Sarasvati's disease (in the biomedical sense), instead of being the singularly targeted enemy against which the forces of biomedical drugs are unleashed, becomes an integral part of a much wider healing process, directed at relieving Sarasvati of a far more profound state of "dis-ease" arising from "the depths of poverty, ignominy, and despair." And the goddess who had once, during

* *Acknowledgements.* The essays by Bhattacharyya, Claus, Daniel, Pugh, and Rhodes are revised versions of papers read in November, 1980, at the IXth Annual Wisconsin Conference on South Asia, in Madison, Wisconsin. The Panel in which these papers were read was entitled "South Asian Medical Systems," and was organized by Robin Gelb and Al Pach, whose help is gratefully acknowledged. We thank Egnor, Hahn, and Ewing for consenting to contribute their essays to this volume. We owe a special word of thanks to McKim Marriott, who served as chairperson and discussant at the original panel and whose perspicuous comments were of great help.

the now extinct epidemics of smallpox, favored the poor, the demographically crowded, and the dietetically "unclean," continues to live in and for the struggle of the downtrodden, today, in the context of an endemic disease, tuberculosis. The subtle changes in definition of the goddess' role, the shifts in the consequences of demographic realities, the paradoxes of love and destruction, all these and more, find brilliantly crystallized expression in the travails and triumph of Sarasvati, the servant of the goddess.

Claus' study of Tulu spirit possession emphasizes a theme which resonates in various ways through the other essays, namely, that spirit possession is a religious phenomenon and a complex mode of personal experience which cannot be adequately described or explained as a medical phenomenon in the biomedical sense. In his accounts of possession, Claus introduces the notion of "disarticulation." There is an articulated and a disarticulated way of being possessed. The latter is a state of distress, of discomfort, of disequilibrium; the former, one of ease, honor, and equipoise. When the possession is an articulate one, there is an obvious measure of grace manifest in speech as well as body movement. And when such an equilibrated relationship has been established, there is no need for exorcism.

There is quite another kind of "disarticulation" recorded in Rhodes' essay. Her fascinating case study concerns a young Sinhalese woman who has a history of miscarrying her pregnancies. In the usual fashion, help and advice is sought from diverse sources, biomedicine included. One crucial piece of advice and prescription comes from a ritual specialist who enjoins her to perform a certain ritual if she is to have a healthy child. For lack of money and other practical reasons the performance of the ritual is postponed. In the meantime, a healthy child is born. The ritual, which assured her of a safe delivery is performed, but three months after the birth of the child. Here Rhodes points out an interesting disarticulation in the temporal sequence. By disengaging the ritual from the strictly temporal linearity of cause and effect, problem (barrenness) and solution (ritual), not only are two dimensions of time created (as Rhodes rightly points out) but two dimensions of space are formed as well. The latter is the equivalent of two fields of significance. The first, the more delimited field of significance, is the patient's inability to conceive. But with the unfolding of events this field comes to occupy the central, but umbral, region of significance. The second dimension is the wider, the more illuminated one. This implicates not merely the problem of barrenness but wider social relationships as well. A unilinear, unitemporal dimension would have inhibited this wider perspective on a state of being ill, obscuring the "situational configuration" which constitutes the patient's problem.

Bhattacharyya compares Freudian psychoanalysis with the form it took in the context of Bengali culture and in the imagination of Girindrasekhar Bose. In the Indian transform, "wish" takes the place of "id," and the "wish" is no longer an individually bounded instinct but an environmentally determined drive. And again, unlike in Freudian psychoanalysis, motivational forces of the wish are not directed at satisfying the id but at "achieving a changed adaptation to the environment.'' Psychoanalysis, unlike earlier therapies, locates therapy in a dialogue. And yet, its locus classicus remains in the individual. Not so in the Indian version: psychoanalysis has had to shift its grounds in order to incorporate the ''environment'' as an integral part of the structure and dynamics of the psyche to a degree that orthodox psychoanalysis would never have done. In addition, Bhattacharyya's discussion points up two ways of achieving quiescence: desires must either be satiated or they must be transcended. And Hinduism provides guidelines as to who may (when and how) satisfy or transcend desire and the suffering it brings with it.

Ewing's study of Muslim pirs in Pakistan and their role as healers once again points out the anomaly of the individual- and disease-centered approach to suffering which is characteristic of biomedicine. The pir's followers consult him on a wide range of problems, and he uses various methods of treatment, such as blowing on the client and writing amulets based on ''luminous knowledge'' associated with the names and attributes of God. Clients seek this knowledge from the pir, which settles on their problems like a calming mantle and shapes itself to their contours. In his performance of exorcism rituals, the pir exorcises the jinn, that is, the afflicting spirit, by the use of spells which operate simultaneously in two domains—the spiritual and the corporeal.

If it is granted that none of the essays are limited to an individual-centered notion of health, then surely, Pugh's essay goes the furthest to make this point. Astrological discourse delimits four mutually coincident aspects of the person—body, mind, and two social aspects of family and community relationships. These four aspects of the person, along with their configurative arrangements in ''personal situations,'' are seen to constitute an important source of conceptual and experiential order in astrological counseling, which deals with a broad and seemingly disparate array of life problems. Pugh points out that the analysis of the broad compass of problems taken up in astrological counseling requires an interpretative perspective whose terms and ultimate theoretical aims do not derive from nor point back to the phenomenon of sickness but rather work from and toward problematic experiences in the life of the person. Furthermore, we find that in this ''astrological hermeneutics'' in which astrologer and client are involved, the ''final'' patterns of relationships among planets, kinsmen, body parts, karmic actions, etc., are not charted by the monological projections of the astrologer and his astrology but by a discourse that is designed as a dialogue, or even a polylogue.

It must not be construed from what has been said thus far and from what is to be said better in the following essays that the ''person'' with his or her distinct problems and existential pains becomes distantiated, diluted, and munisculized by all the inter-, extra-, and trans-personalizations take place in South Asian thought. On the contrary, personal problems are situated in wider contexts which give them greater significance and urgency than were they to have been contained within the confines of a skin-bound individual. ''Situations'' form an essential framework for the conceptualization of the vicissitudes of personal experience, reflecting an articulation among the aspects of the person which goes to constitute the rhythm of life itself and the forms of order and disorder which it manifests (see Pugh 1981). And many of the differences between South Asian systems of healing and thought and those of biomedicine are traceable to the difference in the conceptualization of boundaries by these two systems (see Daniel 1984).

Daniel's essay makes this point most vividly. If there is one ethnographic context among those recorded in the following essays that comes closest to treating the patient as a completely autonomous individual, much like a patient in a doctor's office at Massachusetts General, it is the patient of a Siddha physician. There is very little verbal dialogue that goes on. No invocation of planets are involved and no concern about kinsmen, spirits, or divinities expressed. But even in this highly individualized encounter, the boundary is crossed in the reading of the pulse. Daniel tells us that the Siddha physician diagnoses the patient's condition only when his own pulse pulsates confluently with that of the patient, bringing about a crucial and significant neutralization of the boundary that separates patient and physician.

Daniel's concluding essay also re-presents and recapitulates in semeiotic terms the theme of suffering as a function of disarticulation. The sign relationship that is capable of expressing the greatest degree of articulation is the icon. The icon is a sign in which the object and the representamen have some quality in common. When iconicity is increased to its limit, identity is achieved and the very difference between sign and object is masked, neutralized, or annihilated. Iconicity is the only sign that allows for this possibility. And it is not surprising that the iconic function has a very pervasive and significant presence in South Asian thought in general and in systems of healing in particular. Healing begins, when the problems of the supplicant becomes iconic with the understanding and wisdom of the astrologer or the pir, when the possessed and the possessor become one, when the desirer consumes desire, when time maps onto space, and when physician becomes, for one brief moment, the patient.

REFERENCES

DANIEL, E. Valentine
    1984   *Fluid Signs*: Being a Person the Tamil Way. Berkeley: University of California Press.
OBEROI, J.S.
    1978   *Culture and Science*. New Delhi: Oxford University Press.
PUGH, Judy F.
    1981   Person and Experience: The Astrological System of North India. Ph.D. dissertation, University of Chicago, Dept. of Anthropology.

Contributions to Asian Studies, Vol. XVIII

Rethinking "Illness" and "Disease"

ROBERT A. HAHN*

University of Washington, Seattle, U.S.A.

Our natures are the physicians of our diseases.

Hippocrates

By freeing ourselves from ethnocentric and "medicocentric" views, we may begin to recognize important issues that thus far have been systematically ignored.

Kleinman, Eisenberg, and Good (1978: 251)

A DISTINCTION BETWEEN ILLNESS and disease has recently been elaborated (Feinstein 1967; Fabrega and Manning 1972; Kleinman, Eisenberg, and Good 1978; Frankenberg 1980; Young 1982) to describe the contrast between the perspectives, or worldviews, of patient and physician, and to place these perspectives in sociocultural context. The distinction has begun to broaden the concerns of physicians in practice; it has served also in the formulation of a theory of disease and healing more fully conscious of the importance of psyche and society. It thus enhances the comparison of medical systems across cultural boundaries. A comparative history of this contrast (e.g., Foucault 1973) would chart the unfolding of the healing relation in human history, accounting for the varied forms of distance and engagement between two parties.

Yet, while the illness-disease distinction has been a fruitful one, its recent formulation has been problematic. The distinction has been made inconsistently from work to work, and even within works. Moreover, while attempting to break away from the narrow and exclusive principles of the biomedical conception of Western societies to achieve a truly comparative medical anthropology, recent formulations still bear the impress of this biomedical ideology, including a mind-body dualism, an ascription of primacy to the biological over the

* *Acknowledgments.* I would like to thank the members of a seminar (Dan Blumhagen, Noel Chrisman, Valentine Daniel, Charles Keyes, Arthur Kleinman, Marjorie Muecke, and Gary Rosen) with whom some of these ideas were first discussed in 1980, following seminar notes I presented then.

psychological and the social, and a radical contrast between the "knowledge" of biomedical practioners and the "belief" of patients everywhere and of traditional non-Western healers.

Inconsistencies in this literature may derive from a profound ambivalence inherent in the anthropological quest—the desire to develop a framework which is strong enough to enable the comparative comprehension of others, yet sufficiently susceptible or open to embrace the integrity of those others' own comprehensions. An imperative inherent in much of medical anthropology—the tension between the acute immediacy of a patient's suffering and the chronic finitude of our capacities to know and treat—may also have impeded the development of a consistent distinction.

In this essay I begin an exploration of the conceptual basis for a distinction between illness and disease. I first analyze prominent formulations of the distinctions which have been presented over the past twenty-five years, and I highlight the premises and values underlying these formulations. My analysis is thus a cultural review of medical anthropological thought. I then propose an alternative formulation, providing a more self-consistent comparative framework. The framework balances the universalistic and ethnocentric tendencies of biomedicine with the relativistic and solipsistic strains of phenomenological anthropology; it recognizes the utility of combining biomedical and non-Western conceptions in the development of an essentially comparative epistemology.

The separation between healer (or physician) and patient marked by the terms "disease" and "illness" is enmeshed within a far wider semantic net. Disease is associated with the organic, with the objective, with signs, and with therapy. Illness is associated with the functional, with the subjective, with symptoms, and with care and support. The former moiety is the rational core of medicine—its science, according to its own practitioners; the other, the residual moiety, is the lesser half, problematic and often acknowledged reluctantly and with ambivalence—the art. This semantic network spans the breadth of the medicine of its origins, touching its principal participants, the forms of its pathology, their semiotics, and the prominent responses to them.

The present inquiry has far broader implications as well (see Hahn 1982). It raises the question of pathology as a matter of universal, value-free biological event or of locally determined suffering and failure of purpose. It thus poses the problem of the fundamental work of clinical medicine. It touches also the nominalist-realist contention regarding the nature of events (or things or processes) and labels for them, a contrast (strangely) labeled in the historical and philosophical literature (e.g., Caplan et al. 1981) as one between "physiological" and "ontological"—the hoary problem of reification. The inquiry here thus reaches also anthropological and medical questions about knowledge of disease and suffering, a (bogus yet symbolically charged) tension between science and art, the hard and the soft, and the matters of methodological and moral individualism. The topic of this essay thus branches out to raise questions about human nature, the nature of suffering, its production and relief, and human knowledge of others.

The distinction between illness and disease has a venerable history in Western medical thought. In his well-known statement in *The Epidemics*, Hippocrates proclaimed that "the art consists in three things—the disease, the patient, and the physician. The physician is the servant of the art, and the patient must combat the disease along with the physician" (Hippocrates 1886 I (2,5: 300)). Hippocrates apparently considered fixed diseases to manifest themselves differently in individual hosts under varying environmental situations, described (in translation) as "constitutions." Hippocrates took as significant a great variety of environmental and personal characteristics:

> ... from the constitution, both as a whole and with respect to the parts, of the weather and of each region; from the custom, mode of life, practices, and ages of each patient; from talk, manner, silence, thoughts, sleep or absence of sleep, the nature and time of dreams, pluckings, scratchings, tears; from the exacerbations, stools, urine, sputa, vomit, the antecedents and consequents of each member in the succession of diseases, and the abscessions to a fatal issue or a crisis, sweat, rigor, chill, cough, sneezes, hiccoughs, breathing, belchings, flatulence, silent or noisy, hemorrhages, and hemorrhoids. From these things must we consider what their consequents also will be (Hippocrates 1923 I [3,23]: 181).

As we know from his persistent Oath, Hippocrates also regarded the art of medicine as the exclusive domain of professionals who were obliged to dispense their art in a highly moral fashion to patients, and to transmit their knowledge only to other physicians.

Two millenia after Hippocrates, the medical theorist Thomas Sydenham still held the Greek founder in reverence. Sydenham, best remembered for his realistic, "ontological" postion, sought to lay out a firm classification of the species of disease affecting mankind. He asserted:

> ... it is necessary, in describing any disease, to enumerate the peculiar and constant phenomena apart from the accidental and adventious ones: these last-named being those that arise from the age or temperament of the patient, and from the different forms of medical treatment. It often happens that the character of the complaint varies with the nature of the remedies, and that symptoms may be referred less to the disease than to the doctor. ... Outlying ·forms of disease, and cases of exceeding rarity, I take no notice of. They do not properly belong to the histories of disease. No botanist takes the bites of a caterpillar as a characteristic of a leaf of sage (Sydenham 1981: 147-148).

Diseases were constant despite their apparently varying manifestations. Sydenham combined a higher rationality which implicitly enabled him to separate the essential from the manifest disease, with an empiricism which shunned causal theorizing.

> ... and to prove that those remote and ultimate causes in the determination and exhibition of which the vain speculations of curious and busy men are solely engaged, are altogether incomprehensible and inscrutable; and that the only causes that can be known to us, and the only ones from which we may draw our indications of treatment, are those which are proximate, immediate, and conjunct (Sydenham 1981: 149).

Feinstein on Illness and Disease

Contemporary discussions of this contrast refer to the seminal work of medical theorist Alvan Feinstein (principally 1967). While Feinstein cites the conceptualizations of both Hippocrates and Sydenham in this reflective study, he was not then aware of intellectual precedents for this distinction (personal communication 1982). Feinstein distinguished disease from host from illness as "three types of data":

> For each patient who undergoes treatment, a clinician observes at least three types of data. The first type of data describes a *disease* in morphologic, chemical, microbiologic, physiologic, or other impersonal terms. The second type of data describes the *host* in whom the disease occurs. The description of the host's environmental background includes both the personal properties of the host before the disease began (such as age, race, sex, and education) and also the properties of the host's external surroundings (such as geographic location, occupation, and financial and social status). The third type of data describes the *illness* that occurs in the interaction between the disease and its environmental host. The illness consists of clinical phenomena, the host's subjective sensations, which are called "symptoms," and certain findings, called "signs," which are discerned objectively during the physical examination of the diseased host. When the diseased host seeks medical attention, he becomes a patient, and the clinician's work begins (Feinstein 1967: 24-25).

These definitions are indicative, though not altogether clear. Illness seems to be the manifestation of the disease and its "environmental host." Host-free diseases thus seem to encounter disease-free hosts to produce together illness. These three entities seem to be thing-like rather than event-like or process-like, though the interaction of the first two things seem to produce the third. Illness products consist of clinical phenomena of two sorts: symptoms, that is, the host's subjective sensations, and signs, "certain findings ... which are discerned objectively during the physical examination ..." (Feinstein 1967: 24-25). It is at least possible that laboratory findings from the products (e.g., blood or urine) or activity (e.g., respiration or treadmill testing) might be included as signs, since they would be regarded as objectively discerned from physical examinations. (But see below.)

The host is the patient, or person for whom the disease becomes a perhaps unwanted guest. Feinstein includes as characteristics of the host's environmental background both pre-disease personal characteristics and external circumstances. Not mentioned as part of the host are properties other than personal ones; notably missing are physiological characteristics, which are thus presumably impersonal. When struck by disease, the host manifests an illness whose features include disturbed physiological properties; it is unclear into what realm should fall those undisturbed physiological properties of the pre-disease host.

Paradoxically, disease is the most ambiguous term of Feinstein's triad. Three distinctive alternative interpretations are each consistent with a part of Feinstein's analysis:

Disease₁: A disease is a discrete form with characteristic properties (and perhaps secondary, contingent features) which are manifested in host patients in symptomatic and significant presentations which vary according to variation in the host. Diseases are thus Platonic forms.

Disease₂: The impersonal, that is the non-psychological, non-social, and non-environmental, or, in positive terms, the physiological features of persons, or only of patients, constitute the disease. Disease$_2$ is thus the delimited, discrete part of the patient's body which is disturbed.

Disease$_3$: It may be that signs are objectively evident (to the physician) on first, direct (physical) examination, while less direct assessments from x-rays and cellular analyses are the elements of Disease$_3$. Thus Feinstein writes, "The data that describes the disease can often be obtained by examining the patient's fluids, cells, tissues, excreta, roentgenograms, graphic tracing, and other derivative substances" (Feinstein 1967: 25). Elsewhere (Feinstein 1979), he defines such seemingly objective, hard data as indicative of "paraclinical entities." These are the rock bottom of disease pathology.

Yet, while this reading of Feinstein's "disease" is plausible in terms of his texts, it is grounded in a dubious qualitative distinction between direct and indirect data, between soft and hard data, and between clinical and laboratory or experimental findings. Feinstein is himself sceptical at the same time as he seeks out the unquestionable physical foundations of disease.

The social distribution of knowledge is important in Feinstein's analysis. Patients may report their personal environmental data, thus subjective, to nurses, secretaries, social workers, and others with little or no clinical training. However, illness, and especially disease, are beyond the abilities of patient and paramedicals, and are properly known only by skilled physicians. Even the subjective symptoms of patients are determined by physicians.

In Feinstein's view, the treatment of patients can be broadly divided into two categories: therapeutic and environmental. Therapy deals with mode of treatment; presumably it is the core of medicine. Environmental decisions concern "the management of the host."

> In the reasoning of therapeutic decision, the patient is a case—a representative instance of disease and illness—for which treatment is chosen after comparison with results obtained in similar previous cases. In the reasoning of environmental decisions, the patient is a unique person for whom each aspect of management must be individualized (Feinstein 1979: 25-26).

The therapeutic core of medicine, Feinstein believes, can and should be essentially reduced to the rationality of science. The environmental handmaiden of medicine is essentially intuitive art. "These components of healing are properties of heart and spirit, of instinct and psyche (which) cannot be easily identified, assessed, or quantified by ordinary methods or reasoning" (Feinstein 1964: 945).

Feinstein's conceptualization might be represented as follows:

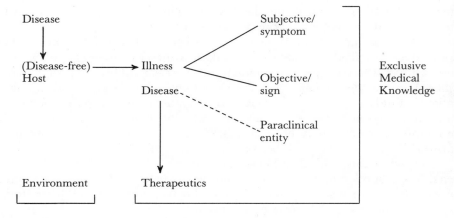

Non-exclusive,
Paramedical Competence
Art

Fabrega and Manning on Disease and Illness, Physical and Mental

Manning and Fabrega argue persuasively for the necessity of combining the approaches of medicine and of sociology to the understanding of human conduct.

> Since human behavior necessarily involves the activation and expenditure of energy that can be traced to organs, systems, and ultimately cells and neurons, and, furthermore, since only behavior of a socially meaningful sort is by definition the concern of *both* medicine and the social sciences, it is surprising that these disciplines do not have a broad framework that encompasses both biological and phenomenological aspects of behavior (Manning and Fabrega 1973: 251-2).

Claiming to build on the work of Feinstein, Engel, and Mechanic, Fabrega and Manning introduce the perspective of phenomenological sociology to the study of events in pathology and healing. Phenomenological sociology (e.g., Berger and Luckmann 1967; Schutz 1967) insists on human conscious experience (of phenomena) as the predominant, if not the only, account of human action.

Fabrega and Manning (1972: 95) find commonalities in the work of Feinstein, Engel, and Mechanic: "All are alike in that the cause of the disease or of the illness is seen as multifactorial, with both genetic and environmental factors playing important roles." The association of Engel and Mechanic with Feinstein is a strange one, for Feinstein's ultimate reality is a paraclinical one, disjoint from the patient's (and the physician's) context; and it is this disjunction to which Engel and Mechanic, and presumably Fabrega and Manning themselves, react strongly.

In rich detail, Manning and Fabrega explore the contrast between the worldviews of biomedicine and non-Western medical systems (Manning and

Fabrega 1973), and between physical ''disease'' and mental ''illness.'' They claim that in mental disturbances, '' ... the self is the illness''; and, since a person's self is largely a social product, the development of a mental illness is also largely a social process. There is a strong hint of mind-body dualism here, a division which contradicts what these authors write elsewhere (e.g., Manning and Fabrega 1973).

In the course of their exploration, Fabrega and Manning formulate a distinction between disease and illness. Yet their usage of these terms contravenes their own definition, rendering their distinction difficult to understand. They define disease and illness as follows:

> Whereas we term the units that the scientific medical system categorizes (that is, diagnoses, interprets, treats) as ''disease,'' we prefer to use the term ''illness'' to depict the socially and culturally patterned entity that members of a group develop and act upon (Fabrega and Manning 1972: 97).

One might infer here that ''group'' refers to anyone not a member of the scientific medical profession, thus patients and non-biomedical practitioners.

In contrast to this definition, Fabrega and Manning write on the previous page (1972: 96) that among ''preliterate'' peoples, ''notions of cause, disease, and illness, which, in the scientific system are logically separated, are fused and condensed.'' Here, instead of taking disease to be what is categorized by the scientific medical system, they seem to relativize the concept of disease itself, suggesting that in preliterate contexts, disease is what the local people think it is. Thus disease is not a condition as conceived by biomedicine, but as conceived by whoever gets ''it'' (or diagnoses ''it''). But then they note (1972: 96-97) that ''in certain ways it can be said that diseases do not ''exist'' in preliterate settings. What do exist, instead, are signs, symptoms, and disabilities that are interpreted and acted upon in terms of the concepts and beliefs of the group.'' Which ''certain ways'' they refer to are uncertain (to me), but now disease may have disappeared altogether (see also Fabrega 1979). But certainly those units referred to by biomedicine persist in such settings (if they are valid in the first place). What is absent is the preliterate thought which matches biomedicine thought. It would seem Fabrega and Manning assume that disease is a conception rather than that to which the conception refers. But what, then, of illness? Is not what they define (Fabrega and Manning 1972: 97) as illness what they describe and then dismiss as disease on the previous page?

Fabrega makes a similar conflation of disease and illness in the summary statement of his book (1974):

> A. Persons can be represented as though they were constituted of a hierarchic array of open and interconnected systems (molecular, chemical, physiological, psychological, social, etc.).
> B. A disease is a person-centered, time-bound, undesirable deviation in the way a person functions (or is characterized by himself and/or by others) in any of these systems (Fabrega 1974: 301).

Here he defines disease in a manner which includes what he has previously distinguished as illness; he then parenthetically dismisses this confusion in the last paragraph of the book:

> H. The use of the behavioral framework of (G) in the study of disease occurrences in various cultural contexts should allow developing a broad sociomedical theory that explains why diseases are produced, what the generic types of disease are and how these are related to each other (this is equivalent to the language and grammar of illness forms discussed in Chapter 5), how diseases happen to develop the culturally distinctive behavioral forms that they do .... (Fabrega 1974: 301).

Why is what was previously distinguished as ''the language and grammar of illness forms'' now casually absorbed into a matter of disease?

The position of Fabrega and Manning on the nature (epistemology) of biology and the ontology of its conditions, e.g., disease, is also unclear. Their assertions range from the a-cultural to the phenomenological. On the one hand, they write of disease as ''... altered functioning of the body as determined by direct evaluation of biological states ...'' (Fabrega and Manning 1972: 103), suggesting firm knowledge without cultural mediation. They talk also of ''the sociocultural value of differentiating between the biological bases of these conditions'' (Fabrega and Manning 1972: 109), again suggesting biology as the ultimate grounds. On the other hand, they often place ''biology'' in quotations, noting ''... processes or events that have been termed 'biological' ...'' (Fabrega and Manning 1972: 94). And Fabrega (1974: 10) emphasizes that ''biological processes themselves are interpreted in terms of culturally specific perceptions.'' Thus they note that biology and biomedicine are belief systems. What is unclear is their own belief. They seem both to accept this system as a firm foundation, and to find it wanting.

Difficulties in the nature of biology, society, disease, and illness spread into those of mind and body and their disturbances. Fabrega (1974: 298) writes, as quoted above, of ''open and interconnected systems (molecular, chemical) ....'' The systems approach posits that different levels are simultaneously at work, each having manifestations and consequences in others. Thus an event is not molecular *or* psychological *or* social, etc., but all three at once, that is, molecular *and* psychological *and* social, etc. Each level pertains to an aspect of a common event. But then why, in Fabrega and Manning's analysis, do disease and illnesses become classified as physical *or* mental, and why do physical problems tend to be called diseases, while mental problems become illnesses? The ontology here is unclear. Despite a move to escape the confines of biomedicine, a profound ambivalence lingers on.

Kleinman, Eisenberg, and Good on Disease and Illness

The various formulations of Kleinman, Eisenberg, and Good (e.g., Kleinman 1973; Eisenberg 1977; Kleinman, Eisenberg, and Good 1978; Kleinman 1980; Good and Good 1981) differ in direction from those of Feinstein. The thrust of their movement is a distinction between what is perceived (and conceived and done) by physicians and what is perceived and done by patients. Yet, while the movement has been one in the right direction, it has been severely obstructed by inconsistency if not self-contradiction, and by implicit assumption of the biomedical perspective it seeks to transcend. Here I offer a close critique of this perspective in order to advance concerted movement in the same direction.[1]

Kleinman, Eisenberg, and Good are inconsistent on three fundamental issues: one concerns the nature of disease, another the relation between disease and illness, and a third the nature of illness. These inconsistencies reflect an essential anthropological dilemma and a profound ambivalence toward biomedicine.

First, they are unclear whether they conceive of disease as a fundamental element of biomedical ideology or whether, in addition, this is an ideology to which they subscribe, at least in part. When they write (Kleinman, Eisenberg, and Good 1978: 25), "modern physicians diagnose and treat *diseases* (abnormalities in the structure and function of body organs and systems) ...," are they implying minimally that this is what modern physicians *think* they are doing, or truly what they *are in fact* doing? If these modern physicians only think they are treating diseases, is this because disease is a false or partially false notion, or because, while there are in truth diseases, these physicians are actually treating something else, that is, something other than diseases?

Kleinman, Eisenberg, and Good's statements lead in two contrary directions. Thus the phrases (1978: 251-252), "... abnormalities in the structure and function of body organs and systems," "... complaints without an ascertainable biologic base," and "... the important influences social and cultural factors have in disease and treatment ...," all suggest that the authors believe not only that physicians believe in disease, but that *there are diseases*—that they, the authors, believe in them too. Their belief would seemingly be modified by the position they adopt, a position which insists on the need for a unified disease-illness approach to theory and practice.

But Kleinman, Eisenberg, and Good also take a contrary position, introducing a third generic element into their scheme—"sickness": "Neither disease nor illness should be regarded as entities. Both concepts are explanatory, mirroring multilevel relations between separate aspects of a complex, fluid, total phenomenon: sickness" (1978: 252). Now the term "entity" is ambiguous, but in their fear of reification, these authors seem to move the concepts of disease and illness from the realm of empirical reality into that of explanatory models or ideology. These notions thus refer to ideas rather than to what these ideas are about. The titles of Kleinman's papers such as "Sickness as Cultural Semantics" (1979) and "Medicine as Symbolic Reality" (1973) also suggest a view of disease, illness, and other medical phenomena as ideal or conceptual rather than real phenomena, what the ideas and concepts are about. From such statements, it is unclear what sort of empirical reality these authors support, if any. Indeed there is a tendency among them to advocate a phenomenologial position in which one's own reality is temporarily "bracketed" or forever undermined by one's own relativity. (The inherent contradictions of this epistemology merit fuller treatment elsewhere.) While not explicitly denying biomedical claims, these assertion move toward granting biomedicine cultural status comparable to that of other medicines. Eisenberg (1977: 14) similarly makes a seemingly ambivalent relativistic claim:

> All belief systems (and we must acknowledge that this includes our own) are culture bound. They make little sense out of context despite their persuasiveness to those brought up to share the same frame of reference.

Yet he cautiously mitigates this claim later:

> Models are ways of constructing reality, ways of imposing on the chaos of the phenomenal world. This is not to deny the independent reality of that world but to emphasize that it does not present itself to us organized in the ways we come to view it (1977: 18).

Phenomenological and semantic positions professed in these writings may be reactions to the massive empiricism of biomedicine. Yet they are over-reactions whose conclusions are equally erroneous.

The second topic on which these authors take inconsistent positions is the relation *between* disease and illness. In their first pair of definitions, neither concept is defined in terms of the other. Diseases are abnormalities of bodily structure and function; illnesses are experiences of disvalued states. These are different sorts of "things"; the authors note, "illness and disease, so defined, do not stand in a one-to-one relation" (Kleinman, Eisenberg, and Good 1978: 251). By a definition of this form, and to the extent that either of element "exists," there may be disease with and without illness, and illness with or without disease. At least according to the definition, neither element is primary or causative to the other, though they may be found to be empirically connected.

A second definition differs significantly: "Viewed from this perspective, illness is the shaping of disease into behaviour and experience. It is related by personal, social, and cultural reactions to disease" (Kleinman 1980: 72). Similarly,

> ... disease in the Western medical paradigm is malfunctioning or maladaption of biologic and psychophysiologic processes in the individual; whereas illness represents personal, interpersonal, and cultural reaction to disease or discomfort" (Kleinman, Eisenberg, and Good 1978: 252).

These definitions are paradoxical in first relativizing the notion of disease to the Western medical paradigm and then universalizing disease and giving it primacy—something to which illness is a secondary and culturally variable reaction. By this definition, while there can be disease with ("symptomatic") and without ("asymptomatic") illness, there can be no illness without disease. It is not clear what relation "discomfort" bears to disease, but the insertion of this term obscures or mitigates a clear relation between disease and illness. (See also Kleinman 1978: 887).

In another variant of this second definition, Kleinman (1980: 72) characterizes illness as "... the psychosocial experience and meaning of perceived disease." By adding perception, the scope of this phenomenon is greatly expanded, for perception allows misperception, distortion, even delusion. This makes room for a great variety of purported illness without disease. These are the so-called functional disorders, e.g., somatization disorder, malingering, and conversion disorder, which are often judged present by the absence of "ascertainable biologic base." (In medicine the current inability to ascertain a "biologic base" seems to be thought of as implying absence of biologic base; in this epistemological process, the patient comes to be regarded as deluded, erroneous.)

Kleinman (1980: 74) refers to illness without disease as "abuses of the medical sick role." Here he joins biomedical colleagues in defining appropriate or correct suffering according to biomedical, nosological etiquette. When the patient's illness is other than a reaction to one of these conditions, he or she is thus said to abuse the medical sick role. (While such patients might be socially offensive, it is not clear here where the abuse lies. Part of the offense of these patients is the inability of biomedicine to treat them. Even in psychiatry, which might be sensitive to the complex social psychological origins of such conditions, responsibility is ascribed individualistically to the sufferer. Such patients might be said to suffer a meta-illness—a painful perceptual response to the perceived conditions of illness itself, an illness about illness.)

A third problem in the formulation of Kleinman, Eisenberg, and Good is the nature or ontology of illness. It is a process, a model, an action, reaction or behavior, an experience, or some combination of these? All of these are suggested in the writings of these authors. Again, do *they* believe that there are "illnesses" or only that patients believe themselves to suffer them?

The authors begin by defining illness as "... experiences of disvalued changes in states of being and social function ..." (Kleinman, Eisenberg, and Good 1978: 251; also Eisenberg 1977: 11). Other definitions increasingly remove the locus of the illness from within the person to greater distances outside of him/her, from the phenomenal to the behavioral to the social:

> Illness, on the other hand, signifies the experience of disease (or perceived disease) and the societal reaction to disease. Illness is the way the sick person, his family, and his social network perceive, label, explain, valuate, and respond to disease (Kleinman 1978: 88).

Similarly illness signifies "... personal, interpersonal, cultural *reactions* to disease or discomfort" (Kleinman, Eisenberg, and Good 1978: 252), "... difficulties in living resulting in sickness ..." (Kleinman, Eisenberg, and Good 1978: 252), and "... disruption in an ongoing biosocial matrix" (Eisenberg 1977: 21).

Whatever the ontology of disease and illness in the formulations of Kleinman, Eisenberg and Good, both of these are said to be "aspects of sickness." Here sickness may be equated with disease; or perhaps there is some third phenomenon; or perhaps one may become ill in reaction to one's prior illness (and disease). Ontological problems are multiplied by this pathological compound.

"Sickness," Kleinman writes (1980: 364), "is best regarded as semantic networks (culturally articulated systems) that interrelate cognitive categories, personal experiences, physiological states, and social relationships." Here again the abstraction comes to the fore, its referent all but ignored.

The etiologies of both disease and illness are simultaneously distinct and interrelated in this formulation. Kleinman's pioneering work on *Patients and Healers in the Context of Culture* explores the ways in which illness is affected by both disease and the social and cultural setting in which it occurs. He shows also how illness affects disease processes. He claims (1980: 74) that in chronic "disorders" (sickness, disease, illness, or?) "it may be difficult to distinguish the disease from the illness."

Yet while these two phenomena are thought to affect one another, there is a fundamental etiological difference between them:

> Disease commonly has a typical course and characteristic features that are independent of setting. Illness is always more or less unique. At times we can talk securely about disease *qua* disease, but illness cannot be understood in that way: it can only be understood in a specific context of norms, symbolic meanings, and social interaction (Kleinman 1980: 77).

Here disease and illness are assumed not simply to be models, but to "exist," probably as processes. Universality lends validity to the phenomenon of disease; fluidity may rain doubt upon the integrity of illness.

Yet analysis of phenomena as unique or universal is a matter of the classification and dimensions on which differentiations are made and the availability of explanations to account for dimensions of interest. According to the schema of Kleinman, Eisenberg, and Good, measles is securely the "same" from place to place, while depression varies widely/significantly. (Within biomedicine, decisions are made according to interpretations of statistical knowledge of likelihoods, successes ascribed to the application of principle to instances, and failure to the uniqueness of individuals.)

In the semantic network formulated by these authors, there is an association between versions of sickness, the person for whom it is a version, the principal cause of what is perceived, and its distribution and variability.

	Percipient	Etiology	Distribution	Treatment	Result
Illness	Patient	Culture	Relative	Care	Relief
	Non-Western Healer???				
Disease		Nature/	Universal	Cure	Remedy
	Physician	Biology			

Frankenberg's and Young's Critique

Frankenberg and Young have recently criticized the disease/illness distinction of Kleinman and colleagues for neglecting the power of human society in the production of pathological processes and in the control of their remedy. By focusing on the healer-patient pair, these authors have given insufficient weight to the massive influences of societal order (and conflict). To correct this imbalance Frankenberg and Young introduce an alternative notion of ''sickness.'' Young does not see his position as a radical break from Kleinman, Eisenberg, and Good; he notes that, in contrast to Taussig (1980), he believes the anthropologies of illness (au Kleinman) and of sickness (Frankenberg and Young) share an epistemological framework. The conceptualizations of Frankenberg are as follows:

> In Lusaka, however, as elsewhere, if *disease*, a pathological entity, is to pass through psychological consciousness—*illness*—to social recognition—sickness—it has to be legitimated. Legitimating agents here again (as elsewhere) are organized in a professional or semi-professional way (Frankenberg 1976: 227-228).

> Disease, by which I mean a biological or pathological state of the organism whether or not it is socially or culturally recognized, and whether or not the patient and his/her advisers, lay or professional, are aware of its existence ... illness, by which I mean the patient's consciousness that there is something wrong (about which in disease terms he/she may or may not be technically correct—a lot here of course depends on who is to be the final judge) .... If, on the other hand, we restrict illness to the making individual of disease by bringing it into consciousness we can use sickness to apply to the total social process in which disease is inserted. This will force us to include in the same process of social interaction and historical development the totality of healers, lay and professional, and the totality of distressed (Frankenberg 1980: 199).

And Young (1982), noting similarities and differences with the formulation of Kleinman:

> DISEASE retains its original meaning (organic pathologies and abnormalities). ILLNESS is essentially the same, referring to how disease and sickness are brought into the individual consciousness.

> SICKNESS is no longer a blanket term referring to disease and/or illness. Sickness is redefined as the process through which worrisome behavioral and biological signs, particularly ones originating in disease, are given socially recognizable meanings, i.e., they are made into symptoms and socially significant outcomes .... The path a person follows from translation to socially significant outcome constitutes his sickness (Young 1982: 270).

The insistence of these authors on the ''socialization of disease and illness'' constitutes an important critique; yet their notions are inconsistent in ways which parallel those of Kleinman and colleagues. Moreover, their notion of socialization goes logically too far in excluding illness in the determination of patient choices, and theoretically not far enough in its determination of processes of disease production.

Since they reject the epistemology inherent in biomedical notions of disease, it is surprising that Frankenberg and Young, like some versions of Kleinman, Eisenberg, and Good, take disease notions for granted, as given elements (i.e., ''data'') to which patients react. While they insist that disease (and illness) are socialized and socially legitimated, they seem to assume that disease pre-existed such social events. Frankenberg suggests either that what counts as pathology is determined without regard to culture, or perhaps only that a people may not be aware of what is good or bad for them. Both interpretations are compatible with biomedical thought itself.

Similarly, while noting (Young 1982: 277) that "*all* knowledge of society and sickness is socially determined" and "... medical facts are predetermined by the processes through which they are conventionally produced in clinics, research settings, etc.," Young also takes "disease" for granted, following Kleinman. The phrase, "... organic pathologies and abnormalities," connotes statistical variation from objectively determined norms, empirical and free of culture and value. Young talks (1982: 278) of "levels of morbidity and mortality" and "pathogens and pathogenic situations." Even when he writes (1982: 278) that "... medical practices are simultaneously ideological practices when they justify (a) the social arrangements through which disease, healing, and curing are distributed in society ... and (b) the social consequences of sickness ...," disease itself is not taken to be the focal element of an ideology. Sickness, then, is a process or path—the historical, temporal sequence of events by which pre-social disease states are socialized. Before such times, disease (or diseases) existed in a natural state (or as natural states).

The development (ontogenetic and/or historical?) of illness is similar. Illness, too, is socialized, thus presumably from some presocialized condition. Its conception, gestation, and birth are not discussed. Frankenberg and Young's brief statements differ slightly here. Frankenberg suggests (1976: 227-228) that disease must "... pass through psychological consciousness—*illness*—to social recognition—sickness ...." Incongruous with his Marxist position, individual psychological formulation seems to precede social recognition, and while legitimating forces are social, what they legitimate is a pre-social given.

Young's brief comment leaves room for an alternative view, for his explanation of illness as "... how disease and sickness are brought into the individual consciousness" (1982: 270) allows a more prominent place for social process. The production of illness may be a social event. Young also writes (1982: 280) of healing as "an ideological practice which helps to reproduce the social relations through which illness is made real and both illness and disease are distributed in society ...." (That sickness is also brought to individual consciousness [in Young's definition of illness] is a happening significantly different from the conscientization of disease, for sickness itself is defined as the socialization of both disease and illness.)

A sickness, then, according to Young, is a process for socializing disease and illness, a path a person follows; according to Frankenberg, it is a social recognition of disease and illness. These are strange definitions, quite at odds with standard lexicography. According to common usage, sickness is not a recognition, nor a process for socialization; sickness is not a path, but a pathology, something suffered. While Frankenberg and Young have corrected a view of disease and illness which neglects the powers of society, they, like Kleinman, Eisenberg, and Good, have confused an account of the phenomenon with the phenomenon accounted for.

Both the metaphors (sickness as a path and as process of socialization) and the reiterative definition of illness as "how ... sickness is brought into individual consciousness" (where sickness, in turn, is the socialization of disease and illness) lead Young into terminological trouble. It is unclear what, following these definitions, he means by such phrases as "... social forces help to determine which people get which sicknesses" (1982: 270), or "... when sickness is brought into the clinic ..." (1982: 272), or, "according to Taussig, it is no accident that sickness has become a focus for ideological practice" (1982: 275). By "sickness" here, does he mean disease, illness (either of these is likely) or a path/process of socialization, as follows from his definition (unlikely)? Similarly, what is the meaning of "... Zande medicine did socialize sickness ..." (1982: 275)? Sickness, by his definition, is socialized disease and illness.

There is another confusion. When Young writes (1982: 271) "that *sickness* rather than illness determines the choice and form of many clinical interventions, transactions, etc.," he suggests, I believe, that social forces cause such choices and forms, and that interests and perspectives other than the patient's may take the fore. But why does the causal power of sickness (a social process) exclude the causal power of illness? Sickness is illness made social. Young's assertion again suggests that illness exists in a presocialized state which is past when the patient makes "choices."

The merit of these authors is to add a certain social perspective to the notions of disease and illness. As I understand it, by socialization they mean: (1) the [social] legitimation of nosological and other categories, and of etiological theory, (2) the social production of such knowledge, (3) the distribution in time and space of susceptibility to pathological conditions, and (4) of resources for treatment in various forms, including (5) the ways in which consociates respond to these conditions. They regard the concern of illness theorists with efficacy as only one element in a broader concern with the social distribution of pathology, health, and belief.

Yet, despite their socialized view, Frankenberg and Young seem ambivalent, like Kleinman, Eisenberg and Good, about biomedicine and its focal "disease." They define disease as do biomedical practitioners, and, while they talk of its legitimation and its socialization, they seem to take it both as having presocialized ontological status and as being securely legitimated. Despite their assertion that they will be "forced" "to include in the same process of social interaction and historical development the totality of the distressed," their social process of sickness is built upon biomedical foundations. Young productively pursues the compromises made when "Rational Men Fall Sick," but not when rational men heal. Patients know; physicians really know.

Disease and Illness Revised

I propose a revised medical anthropological framework in which the standard order of disease and illness is stood upon its head. I begin with the pan-human phenomenon of suffering. Suffering is understood by suffering patients as "illness," by biomedical practitioners as "disease," and by healers and thinkers of other traditions as "disorders" of different sorts. The proposed framework is pluralistic and ecumenical, egalitarian and democratic; it is eclectic and reflexive. It strongly doubts the exclusive validity of any one perspective, and explicitly seeks to encompass the notions and theories of different systems in a move toward a more comprehensive medical anthropology. It restores to pathology its original sense as the science and treatment of pathos, i.e., suffering.

Suffering is found universally in human societies and among their members. Most of us find this most unfortunate. There are mythical accounts of days before the fall, and other hopeful accounts of future release from such a fate. Suffering is understood and encountered in widely varying fashions, again by different societies and among their members. It is thought of as self-inflicted or inflicted by another—perhaps a spirit or a force. It is held to be lodged in body, mind, or self, or more widely dispersed within the web of relations among the beings of the world. It may be accepted passively as human nature or social obligation; or it may be actively resisted as an obstacle to human fulfillment. I mean only to crudely suggest the dimensions and variations which may be found, rather than to propose an exhaustive paradigm of the forms of suffering.

I propose three ideal-typical ideologies of suffering, that is, conceptual, epistemological, aesthetical and ethical, affective and theoretical, more or less coherent system of ideas, understandings, or models of suffering: *Illness-ideologies* (the perspectives of the sufferers), *Disease-ideologies* (the specific perspectives of biomedical practitioners), and *Disorder-ideologies* (the varied perspectives of traditional, non-Western healers). These cuttings and lumpings are crude, to be sure; they point to significantly distinctive perspectives on the matter (or spirit) of suffering. They are ideal-types in that they are seldom found in isolated, pure form; in various cultural and historical settings, these ideologies have significantly influenced each other and continue to do so, in the confrontation of institutional and societal forces and in the clinical encounters of patients and healers (Helman 1978; Blumhagen 1980).

In a gross fashion, ideologies of illness, disease, and disorder may be differentiated by the spaces—physical, personal, social, environmental, and cosmological—in which they localize the problem of suffering and its resolution. This more or less exclusive differentiation may be mapped as follows:

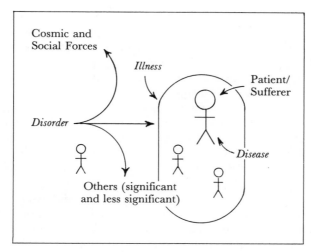

Universe/Cosmos

Disease is located with the body, at or beneath the skin, and most often below the mind. This is thus the ideology called biomedicine. Illness ideologies ascribe suffering and its causes to the sufferer's person and his/her immediate environment; it thus includes the body, but reaches beyond as well. Disorder ideologies localize (or disperse) suffering to persons as the foci much broader social and/or cosmological nexi and forces.

Whereas illness ideologies begin with the patient's suffering, referring to a failure to achieve a valued state, disease ideologies are commonly phrased in terms of either ''maladaptations'' or ''abnormalities in the structure and function of body organs and systems'' (Kleinman, Eisenberg, and Good 1978: 251). Notions of ''maladaptation'' and ''abnormality'' bear a connotation of empirical assessment, free from value-judgment. ''Abnormality'' suggests deviation from a statistical norm. Insofar as the frameworks of the authors I have reviewed are oriented toward disease, defining other terms as reactions to disease, they may accept such connotations (see also Boorse 1975). I would argue strongly that this represents a false consciousness, an erroneous epistemology; for even the medicalized notions of suffering (that is, pathology) which are embodied in the ''disease'' nosology are originally grounded in human value, largely cultural phenomena.

Rather than ascribing primacy to disease, and then regarding illness as secondary—the patient's reaction to disease, the framework I propose gives primacy to illness—the patient's understanding of his/her suffering. Thus, while the patient's theory may be partly or largely mistaken, it is his/her experience of suffering which engenders the whole medical enterprise. The sufferer's judgment rather than that of biomedicine defines the *underlying problem*. It is this fundamental problem which disease-, disorder-, and illness-ideologies address, and to which they minister. Yet, while ascribing primacy to suffering, my framework regards illness-, disease-, and disorder-ideologies as ontologically equivalent—all ideologies.

All ideologies are socially constructed elements of more or less coherent systems. Ideologies divide up and reconnect the world according to local principles and interests (and conflicting interests). An ideology is one picture (or sketch) among numerous alternatives. Disease-, illness-, and disorder-ideologies, for example, are explicitly and implicitly taught and differentially distributed within (and among) societies. They are real in their existence in human minds and thought, and in their effects—a partial causality—in human action. While these and other effects may increase the likelihood that a reality believed in is true, belief does not logically imply anything about the reality believed.

I draw a sharp distinction between an *ideology* and what the ideology is about, its *referents*, its *reality*. An ideology may be hallucinatory, deluded, false or partially false. But I am not using "ideology" in the sense of critical Marxism—false consciousness, by definition. An ideology may also be valid here and there; it may thus be better than other ideologies here and /or there. Yet, at the extremes, ideologies may exist even if what they claim is entirely false, or even incoherent, thus when their referent realities do not exist; realities persist despite ideologies.

Within such extremes, ideologies and their referents interact in ways which are of great significance in processes of pathology (illness, disease, and

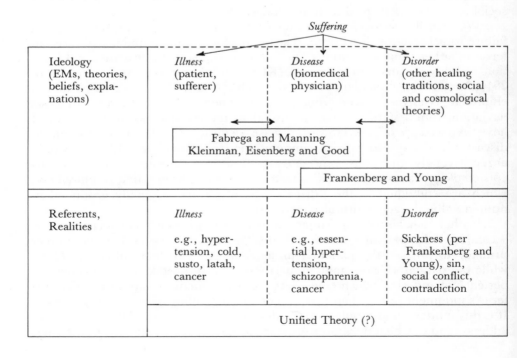

disorder) and healing (perhaps, care/healing, cure, and reordering). (See Hahn and Kleinman 1983.) Ideology affects the world about which it purports, while this world may constrain ideological constructions of it. There is a good deal of evidence that belief affects, and may even effect what it is about. The consequences range from voodoo death, in which fear and expectation of death leads to death, to the placebo phenomenon, in which the hope and expectation of healing lead to healing. While it is essential to distinguish the model from what it models, both may have like outcomes. Cancers and models of cancer may both kill, though they do so by different means.

Suffering-Ideologies and Their Referents

Referent realities reciprocally affect ideologies by a society-wide form of reality testing, a natural selection of belief. The world objects to severe misconceptions of it. Severely misguided ideologies lead their proponents to self-destruction. More objective belief may lead proponents astray, and may be adjusted or rectified when or if noted. Life has features of an experiment in which belief may be persistently tested.

Whether and which (referent) illnesses, diseases, and disorders *exist* or are *real* is a question of theoretical and empirical research. We look for how much each of these proposed notions explains in what we observe, and we examine how this notion hangs together with others that we hold. Perhaps a fundamental tenet of anthropology, we may conjecture that no formulation is likely to be exclusively valid, and that most are likely to contribute something to our understanding. The nineteenth century germ theory of disease added enormous strength to our understanding of certain kinds of diseases, while continuing to lead us astray on others. Some of the referent entities or processes of each ideology—illness, disease, and disorder—give good explanations for the manifestations and shapes of human suffering. We must build a framework which takes each alternative, informant framework seriously enough to encompass its understandings, while not taking each framework (including our own) so seriously as to exclude other possibilities. To move cautiously forward, we need a reasonable place to stand.

Kleinman (1980: 377-378) strongly urges that "In analyzing and comparing clinical categories and situations, it is essential that anthropological investigations do not accept the biomedical paradigm as the appropriate theoretical frame for describing and interpreting them." One might first note that by defining illness as a reaction to disease (or perceived disease), and by suggesting that illness without disease is abuse of the medical sick role, Kleinman has himself accepted the biomedical paradigm despite his anthropological quest. But then, while we would not want to accept the biomedical paradigm whole-hog, in its exclusive presumptions, nor would we want to entirely reject this paradigm. We take biomedicine for what it is worth. Substantial parts of its nosology, theory, and research methodology are essential elements for an (anthropological) exploration of suffering and healing. We must only assure that the paradigm be broadened to encompass the complementary under-standings of illness and disorder, and that perverse forms of suffering, perhaps meta-sufferings (the suffering about suffering, as in hypochondria), not be regarded as the sufferer's abuse. We may then wish to find abuse in the wider sources of the sufferer's presentation.

In the framework I am proposing, the events which happen to persons (or in which persons participate) have multiple *aspects*, for example, physical, chemical, physiological, psychological, anthropological, and environmental. Each aspect forms a system of interacting elements (Brody and Sobel 1979). The systems are more or less open, since the interaction of their elements is both influenced by and itself influences phenomena which are not in that system. The aspects are sometimes said to form a hierarchy—in the order listed above; the order to the levels may accord with the size of the elements (physical ones smaller than physiological ones), or, more probably, their greater in-clusiveness. Chemical elements include (or are composed of) physical ones, physiological elements include chemical ones, etc. The ordering however, is not clear, and there remains a difficulty regarding relations between levels—a tension between reductionism (the principle that higher-level aspects can be fully reduced or explained in terms of lower-level aspects) and emergentism (the contention that the properties of higher-level systems can not be explained in terms of lower-level systems, and that higher-level systems have emergent properties). A systems approach has not been fully worked out. Nevertheless, I believe it provides a framework appropriate to an understanding of multiplex human phenomena.

Of particular merit in the systems approach is the avoidance of dualisms, triadisms, or worse pluralisms. The systems approach posits interactions be-tween phenomena and the different levels by which they may be analyzed. It is thus a synthetic framework. Instead of asking whether some phenomenon or event is physiological *or* psychological *or* social, it assumes the phenomenon or event to have at the same time physiological, psychological, *and* social aspects. Disciplines do not have exclusive terrains of exploration; they share fields, looking only at different aspects.

Thus the medical division between psychosomatic and non-psychosomatic, presumably somatosomatic, and perhaps somatopsychic and psychopsychic diseases, is excessively clearcut. It suggests a falsehood—that one event (or complex of events) which is psychic and not somatic causes another event (or complex) which is somatic but not psychic. In the framework I propose, any human event is likely to have both such aspects at once, along with others. This brings into question other divisions within biomedicine—be-tween organic and functional and between physical and mental diseases.

Questionable also is the possibility of illness with or without disease, with or without disorder. I discern two questions here: First, in the current state of our knowledge of illness, disease, and disorder, can one of these be found to ex-ist without the other; and what permutations are found? Second, as our understanding of illness, disease, and disorder improves, will further connec-tions (or separations) be found?

Certainly, by our current understandings of illness, disease, and disorder, each of these may exist in isolation, and all permutations are possible. Hypertension is most often an asymptomatic disease, one without an illness (although when medically diagnosed as hypertensive, people thus become patients, commonly believing themselves to have hypertension, an illness [Blumhagen 1980]). Similarly, early cancerous growths may be asymptomatic, thus unlikely to be illnesses; indeed, it is questionable at what point they become diseases—at the first malignant division or at first diagnosis?

The so-called functional diseases, e.g., conversion disorder and hypochondria, are commonly cited as illness without disease. Disorder may likewise exist without recognized disease or illness, as when social disorder is not felt to cause suffering. (Recently the ideology of "stress" has brought disorder closer to disease and illness, though in paradoxical fashion [Young 1980].)

I would suggest, however, that as our understanding of illness, disease, and disorder increases, it will be found that manifestations of any of these in isolation, that is, in the absence of the others, is less likely. It will increasingly be recognized that the occurrence of an illness does correspond to a disease (or several) perhaps not previously recognized, and to a disorder (or several) perhaps also not previously recognized, and so on. The classification of diseases as organic and functional (in which biomedical psychiatry's Diagnostic and Statistical Manual of Mental Disorder is founded) or physical and mental will be superceded. Functional diseases, so classified because of absent "discernible organic base," will be found to have at least organic correlates, and means by which social and symbolic processes are embodied. Improved understanding of illness may come about by increased patient awareness of pathological processes. We know that people learn to attend to or ignore such processes through interactions with others (Frankenberg and Young's "sickness"). By means of these same processes and extensions of them, such as biofeedback, or perhaps sociofeedback (e.g., Jordan 1977), people may become more aware of bodily and environmental (natural and social) events which affect their health. Further research into disease and disorder, for example, in social and psychiatric epidemiology, should similarly reveal the correspondences of these with each other and with illness. Those illnesses classified as abuses of health care should be explained, and the conception of health care expanded to disperse and redress the sources of abuse. Divisions between these ideologies and their referents may become more apparent than real.

The proposed framework should be more appropriate to comparative research. It is neither exclusively nor principally based in biomedical notions of disease, but rather in the pan-human phenomenon of suffering. Nor does it divide up body, mind, society, and universe as exclusive domains with exclusive disciplinary knowledge. For these characteristics, the proposed framework more closely approximates the systems it may study, for example, the medical systems of Asia; the possibilities for communication are thus enhanced. Ideologies of illness, disease, and disorder are accounts for the phenomenon of suffering. They may conflict, and they may be reconciled. In this reconciliation, we may better know and respond to human processes of suffering and healing.

NOTE

1 Kleinman has significantly altered his position on the "illness"—"disease" distinction in a recent analysis of "neurasthenia" in China (Kleinman 1982; see also Kleinman 1983). In this study he gives primacy to the understanding of the patient who enters medical settings with an "illness" which is then transformed into a "disease" by biomedical practitioners.

REFERENCES

BERGER, Peter L. and Thomas LUCKMAN
    1967   *The Social Construction of Reality*. Garden City, New York: Doubleday.
BLUMHAGEN, Dan
    1980   "Hyper-tension: A Folk Illness with a Medical Name." *Culture, Medicine, and Psychiatry* 4(3): 197-227.
BOORSE, Christopher
    1975   "On the Distinction between Disease and Illness." *Philosophy and Public Affairs* 5: 49-68.
BRODY, Howard and D. S. SOBEL
    1979   "A Systems View of Health and Disease." *In* D. S. Sobel (ed.), *Ways of Health*. New York: Harcourt, Brace and Jovanovich.
CAPLAN, Arthur et al
    1981   *Concepts of Health and Disease*. Reading, Massachusetts: Addison-Wesley.
EISENBERG, Leon
    1977   "Disease and Illness." *Culture, Medicine, and Psychiatry* 1(1): 9-23.
FABREGA, Horacio, Jr.
    1974   *Disease and Social Behavior*. Cambridge, Massachusetts: Massachusetts Institute of Technology Press.
    1979   "Elementary Systems of Medicine." *Culture, Medicine, and Psychiatry* 3(2): 167-198.
FABREGA, Horacio, Jr. and Peter MANNING
    1972   "Disease, Illness, and Deviant Careers." *In* R. A. Scott and J. D. Douglas (eds.), *Theoretical Perspectives on Deviance*. New York: Basic Books.
FEINSTEIN, Alvan R.
    1964   "Scientific Methodology in Clinical Medicine III: The Evaluation of Therapeutic Response." *Annals of Internal Medicine* 61(5): 944-965.
    1967   *Clinical Judgment*. Huntington, New York: Robert E. Krieger.
    1979   "Science, Clinical Medicine, and the Spectrum of Disease." *In* Beeson, Paul B., W. McDermott, and J. Wyngaard (eds.), *Cecil Textbook of Medicine*. Philadelphia: W. B. Saunders.
FOUCAULT, Michel.
    1973   *The Birth of the Clinic*. New York: Vintage Books.
FRANKENBERG, Ronald
    1980   "Medical Anthropology and Development: A Theoretical Perspective." *Social Science and Medicine* 14B(197-207).
FRANKENBERG, Ronald and Joyce LEESON
    1976   "Disease, Illness and Sickness: Social Aspects of Choice of Healer in a Lusaka Suburb." *In* J. B. Loudon (ed.), *Social Anthropology and Medicine*. New York: Academic Press.
GOOD, Byron and Mary-Jo GOOD
    1981   "The Meaning of Symptoms: A Cultural Hermeneutic Model for Clinical Practice." *In* Leon Eisenberg and Arthur Kleinman (eds.), *The Relevance of Social Science for Medicine*. Dordrecht, Holland: Reidel.

HAHN, Robert A.
1982   Review of *Concepts of Health and Disease*, edited by Arthur Caplan, H. T. Engelhardt, and J. J. McCartney. *Medical Anthropology Newsletter*, 14; 1.
HAHN, Robert and Arthur KLEINMAN
1983   "Belief as Pathogen, Belief as Medicine: 'Voodoo Death' and the Placebo Phenomenon in Anthropological Perspective." *Medical Anthropology Newsletter*, 14; 4:3, 16-19.
HELMAN, Cecil
1978   " 'Feed a Cold, Starve a Fever'—Folk Models of Infection in an English Suburban Community and their Relations to Medical Treatment." *Culture, Medicine, and Psychiatry* 2(1): 107-138.
HIPPOCRATES
1886   *The Genuine Works of Hippocrates*. Francis Adams, trans. New York: William Wood.
1923   *Hippocrates*. Vol. 1. W. H. S. Jones, trans. New York: G. B. Putnam's Sons.
JORDAN, Brigitte
1977   "The Self-Diagnosis of Early Pregnancy: An Investigation of Lay Competence." *Medical Anthropology* 1(2): 1-38.
KLEINMAN, Arthur M.
1973   "Medicine's Symbolic Reality." *Inquire* 16: 206-213.
1978   "Concepts and Models for the Comparison of Medical Systems as Cultural Systems." *Social Science and Medicine* 12: 85-93.
1979   "Sickness as Cultural Semantics: Issues for an Anthropological Medicine and Psychiatry." *In* P. Ahmed and G. Coelho (eds.), *Toward New Definitions of Health: Psychosocial Dimensions*. New York: Plenum.
1980   *Patients and Healers in the Context of Culture*. Berkeley: University of California Press.
1982   "Neurasthenia and Depression," *Culture, Medicine and Psychiatry*, 6; 2: 117-90.
1983   "Editor's Note," *Culture, Medicine and Psychiatry*, 7; 1: 97-99.
KLEINMAN, Arthur, Leon EISENBERG, and Byron GOOD
1978   "Culture, Illness, and Care." *Annals of Internal Medicine* 88(2): 251-258.
MANNING, Peter K. and Horacio FABREGA, Jr.
1973   "The Experience of Self and Body: Health and Illness in the Chiapas Highlands." *In* George Psathas (ed.), *Phenomenological Sociology*. New York: John Wiley.
SCHUTZ, Alfred
1967   *Collected Papers*. The Hague: Martinus Nijhoff.
SYDENHAM, Thomas
1981   "Preface to the Third Edition, *Observationes Medicae*." *In* Arthur Caplan et al (eds.), *Concepts of health and Disease*. Reading, Massachusetts: Addison-Wesley.
YOUNG, Allan
1980   "The Discourse on Stress and the Reproduction of Conventional Knowledge." *Social Science and Medicine* B14: 133-146.
1981   "When Rational Men Fall Sick: An Inquiry into Some Assumptions Made by Medical Anthropologists." *Culture, Medicine, and Psychiatry* 5: 317-335.
1982   "The Anthropologies of Illness and Sickness." *Annual Review of Anthropology*. Palo Alto, California: Annual Reviews.

The Changed Mother
or
what the Smallpox Goddess did when there was no more Smallpox*

MARGARET TRAWICK EGNOR

Hobart and William Smith Colleges, Geneva, N.Y., U.S.A.

AMONG THE MANY HEALERS IN MADRAS, some are human and some are not. Some are deities, who rely upon human helpers, as doctors rely upon nurses, to mediate between themselves and their patients, but who are not considered to be in any way commanded or controlled by these human helpers—rather, the reverse is true. And yet, just as nurses do sometimes control the acts of doctors, the human helpers of divine healers are not entirely passive transmitters of the deities' powers.

In the present essay, the evolving relationship between one such human helper and the deity she serves will be described.[1] One realization that I came to in studying this relationship was that Hindu deities are not only symbols or tools which are manipulated by human beings to express certain ideas—such deities are actors, with wills of their own, and to a great extent they do control the lives of their servants, whether the latter are willing or not. A second realization that I made was that deities, despite their wilfulness, are not inflexible. In order to survive, they must change to fit the times, and they do. In the protean environment of South Asian culture, deities, like many other entities, are highly "context variable," and especially when they enter into close relations with particular human beings is this so.[2]

In the city of Madras, healing by deities is a medical genre, like Āyurveda or allopathic medicine, with certain regular features. A deity will choose a human servant, and through possession and dreams will communicate to the chosen one the deity's commands. The chosen servant becomes a vehicle of the

* *Acknowledgments.* The research upon which this essay is based was carried out in 1975-1976 under a fellowship from the Social Science Research Council and in 1980 under a grant from the American Institute of Indian Studies.

deity's power, the servant's house a temple to the deity, and the servant's body the deity's own. The servant's house will be marked as a temple by the symbol of the deity before the doorstep, and the servant's body will be marked by matted hair. Having become established as a professional vehicle of the deity, a priest or priestess, the servant at regular times during the week becomes possessed by the deity. At such times, individuals seeking the deity's help will come to the servant's house. The deity will speak through the servant to each supplicant, and the deity's power, acting through the servant, will solve the supplicants' problems and heal their illnesses.

There is little specialization among deities or their servants in respect to the difficulties treated: physical disease, mental distress, demon possession, loss of objects or persons, family conflicts, legal difficulties, anxiety over examinations—all may be handled in the same healing session. Talk, verbal persuasion, is an important aspect of the healing process. The deity speaking through the servant chastises, reassures, preaches, argues and commiserates with each supplicant as the case warrants. The servant also, before and after the period of possession, talks with the patients and extols the deity's powers. Since many people may be present at a healing session, to be entertained as well as to be healed, acts of healing are very public, and involve the patients' public confession of their problems and sorrows. Personal qualities of the servant are important. The success of an individual servant is in large measure dependent upon the servant's own persuasive abilities.[3]

One of the most important of the healing deities in Madras is the goddess of smallpox, Māriamman. Nearly every Māriamman temple has associated with it a person whom the goddess regularly possesses and through whom she heals and speaks with supplicants. There are also many vehicles of the goddess' healing powers who are not associated with any particular temple other than their own houses and bodies. Although the bulk of those applying to the goddess for aid are poor people belonging to lower castes, her clientele spans all classes. It also includes both sexes, although most of her servants and supplicants in the city of Madras are women. As a healer, and the guiding force behind a large number of individuals who earn part or all of their livelihood by acting as her vehicles, Māriamman competes successfully with other professionalized healing establishments in the city.[4] As a deity, she is on a par with the other major deities of the area in terms of popularity, wealth, and increasingly, status and authority.[5]

An acquaintance with the smallpox goddess in India leads one to ask a number of questions, one of which is, why would people deify a disease? For in cases of smallpox, people say, or used to say, that the disease *is* the mother, and she will be angered by any attempts to combat it. Yet if, for whatever reason, this disease is considered to have its own will, why could it not have been personified as a demon, and a deity with a different identity called in to heal it? In fact, many diseases have been personified as demons in various South Asian traditions, and demons are commonly exorcised with the aid of deities.[6] If it is possible to separate the killing from the healing power, why has it not been done here?

A second question we must ask is, of all the diseases that might have been deified, why was smallpox chosen? There are other diseases—such as malaria, typhoid, cholera, and polio—that have taken an equal or greater toll in India and diseases such as leprosy which are even more dramatically disfiguring. Yet even where such diseases have been personified, they have not in recent times been deified, and major cults have not been centered around them, as has happened with Māriamman.

A third question that arises is, given that smallpox is a deity, why is it a goddess? Why should *this* disease take the form of a female, when so many others—most of the Sinhalese disease demons, the Bengali fever demon Jvarāsur, the Vedic Rudra—are or were male?

And why, given that smallpox is female, is she a mother? Descriptions of the "grace" of the smallpox goddess, of her "maternal love," seem to the Westerner to be laden with irony. The pustules produced by smallpox are called the "pearls" bestowed by the mother, or her "kisses" (*muttu, muttam*). The goddess herself is called the "cool one" (Śītalā) in Hindi and Bengali, and similarly in Tamil her name means "rain mother"—where rain, moisture and coolness are closely associated with concepts of love, pleasure, and compassion.[7] Yet the disease smallpox causes great fever and pain. When someone gets smallpox, therefore, it may be referred to not only as the "grace" of the mother and her "love," but also, as her "rage." She enters the body of a person out of "desire" for them, love for them, but the fever of smallpox is interpreted as the heat of her anger.

A final question that the existence of the smallpox goddess leads us to ask is, what will happen to her, now that smallpox is apparently no longer present in India? It would not be unreasonable to expect some kind of correlation to exist between the popularity of the cult of the smallpox goddess and the severity and frequency of the epidemics that she is thought to cause. Indeed, just such a correlation has been found for certain periods of Indian history, in certain regions.[8] Since smallpox is no longer endemic in India, one might predict that the cult of the smallpox goddess should soon weaken and die.

The eradication of smallpox in the city of Madras has been quite dramatic. As recently as 1958, there occurred the worst smallpox epidemic in at least thirty years, in which 4869 cases and 1260 deaths were reported in Madras city alone[9] (Rao 1972: 176-177). Lesser but still serious epidemics occurred in 1961 and 1963; the very occurrence of major epidemics at these times was ominous, since the epidemic cycle of smallpox throughout the twentieth century normally peaked every fifth year, not every second (Rao 1972: 176ff).

In October 1963, the World Health Organization's National Smallpox Eradication program was initiated in Madras. Each year after that there was a radical reduction in the number of cases reported. In 1970, for the first time, there were no cases reported at all (Rao 1972: 176). In the mid-1970's, a vaccination scar was visible on every left arm, even of servants of the goddess. And though notices were posted throughout the cities and countryside offering large rewards for information leading to the discovery of smallpox cases, no such cases became known.

Yet in the late 1970's, far from being moribund, the cult of the smallpox goddess showed many signs of flourishing good health. I followed the career of one of the servants of the goddess, observing the changes that her life underwent from 1975 through 1976, and again between that time and 1980. Just as the star of the disease was setting this priestess' star had begun to rise. When I first met her, she was still living with her large family in a small mud hut in an area that wealthier people of the neighborhood referred to as "the slum." Here she had lived for a decade. But the house contained many new stainless steel cooking utensils, dozens of expensive saris, and fine jewelry—gifts of devotees of the goddess and of followers of this particular priestess. She also had several head of buffalo, and the herd grew as the months and years passed. By 1980 she had built for herself a new concrete house, and she sponsored yearly neighborhood festivals in honor of the goddess.

This priestess of the goddess Māriamman was only one of many living in Madras, and perhaps her good fortune was unusual. However, as the city expanded, new priestesses of the goddess appeared, and small mud houses with tridents at the entrance, symbol of Māriamman, could be seen where previously there had been none. It seemed that devotion to the goddess, beyond the deeper spiritual and psychological factors which gave rise to it, was also a viable way of earning a living.

More impressive was the growth of a very large temple to Māriamman in Tiruvērkāḍu, a northern suburb of Madras. This had been a small temple, but at the time of my visit it was being completely rebuilt at great expense. With thousands of visitors weekly, lavish month-long festivals, and gorgeous, gilded chariots built by sculptors brought in from distant states, Tiruvērkāḍu had become one of the wealthiest and most glamorous temples in Madras. Previously there had been no large Māriamman temple in all of Tamil Nadu.[10]

Hence the popularity of the smallpox goddess, the number of her devotees and the amount of wealth spent in her worship, does not appear to have been dependent, at least in this modern urban environment, upon the prevalence or even the existence of smallpox itself. If it was not because people feared the disease she might inflict, why then did they worship her?

Sarasvati, the servant of the goddess with whom I worked, spoke of Māriamman as of a loved and admired close friend. With a broad smile and eyes shining, she would relate to visitors anecdotes concerning the goddess. Her tone was one of mingled awe and affection. Once when I was there a small snake crossed the floor of the house. Sarasvati noticed it and cried, "It's her! It's her! You have wanted to see the mother. There she is!" Subsequently, visitors were told of the time that the mother took the form of a beautiful little serpent and danced before the eyes of the questioning American. The snake lived behind another form of the mother, a triangular black stone with gleaming metal eyes and ivory fangs, lying on the floor in the middle of the hut, adorned with garlands of flowers and lemons. Every week, Sarasvati would perform *abhiṣēkham* for the goddess, carefully washing the stone as though it were a real human face, and reapplying its make-up. The goddess also appeared to

Sarasvati in dreams, speaking directly to her; she took Sarasvati's own form, speaking through her to others when Sarasvati became possessed; and she acted invisibly, leading clients to Sarasvati and causing their troubles to be ended. Sometimes it seemed that nothing was not her.

From the beginning of her life, Sarasvati dwelt upon a kind of cultural frontier.[11] She belonged to a low caste family, but her father owned a liquor store and worked for a major newspaper, both occupations made lucrative by the British presence. To own an urban liquor store was to reject high-caste Hindu ideals and to convert one's low-caste status into a modern asset. But with independence and prohibition, this particular avenue of advancement was closed in Tamil Nadu.

At the age of sixteen, "as soon as I came of age," she said, Sarasvati eloped with the chauffeur of a movie actress. The idea of elopement is ancient in Tamil Nadu, but in the twentieth century, "love marriages" are especially associated with Western ideals and values, as are automobiles, chauffeurs, and movie actresses. This world was and remains very much opposed to the world of traditional caste Hinduism, where the power and sexuality of women is active but concealed, and where physical and social mobility are restricted by bonds of a thousand kinds. A person standing on the boundary between those two worlds in any given situation must choose one or the other. It is impossible to have it both ways.

In marrying as she did, Sarasvati chose to defy tradition, yet in other respects, she stood firmly for older values. Even as a child, she had great religious devotion; she visited all the nearby temples frequently, and had no other interest. "I did nothing else," she said. Like many orthodox Hindus, she spurned and ridiculed people who claimed to be possessed by deities, until she herself became possessed by one. After her possession, she continued to support traditional values. She was opposed, for instance, to the ideas of divorce and widow remarriage. She believed that Western women moved easily from husband to husband and she felt that such behavior was wrong.

Just as she swung between the conflicting worlds of Westernized and traditional Madras, Sarasvati swung also between Brahmanical values and the populism of the lower castes. In some respects, her behavior imitated that of very orthodox Brahmans. She bathed several times daily. She did not eat meat, eggs, fish, or sweets. She ate only in her own home, not in other people's houses or in hotels, except for hotels run by Brahmans. She would not eat from a plate, but only from a leaf. All of these restrictions she said the goddess had imposed upon her, yet when the goddess possessed her, she performed animal sacrifices and ate the raw meat.

Although she was unschooled, her speech was highly Sanskritized, and so well did she imitate Brahman dialect that one Madrasi Tamil with a Ph.D. in linguistics, hearing a tape-recording of her speech, thought at first that she must be a Brahman. Yet she disdained any pretensions to high ritual status. "I do not put on wet/ritually pure clothes. I have no Sanskrit Veda. I have no learning," she said. "I have no desire to build a fine house and live in it. To build a house of several stories, to be good and Sanskritic (*samaskirutamāka*), all of that I do not want." Instead, she claimed identity with the poor and despised.

Sarasvati believed that the goddess loved and protected mostly the poor, the uneducated, the members of untouchable castes, and "Tamil women"—all of those who lacked status and external power, but who were internally pure. "The heart must be clean," she said, in order for the goddess to enter it. The goddess entered a person in two ways, through possession and through disease. Sarasvati did not distinguish between the two. "The mother makes pearls [causes pox]. In the person of a child, or in the person of an adult, following her desire she comes; because she feels attracted to someone she comes. She will not come in everyone's person. Ordinarily, the kind of person she likes most is someone of an untouchable group; in their person she has much desire. In their person she will come very often."

The goddess visited the rich also, but not to protect them. The rich and well-educated were too arrogant to have faith, and so when the goddess tested them, they failed and succumbed to disease, while the poor and simple were saved. Sarasvati said,

> A man who has not studied is poor, but he will have that mother's devotion. If someone wants to do research in the world, they can do nothing. But the man with devotion, no one can deceive him. In any life, in any labor, he will have all wisdom. The reason is that he has that mother's grace. Because he has belief, even if ten people come to get him, he can say, Go away. My mother is here to protect me. Those ten people will think he is lying. One of them will say, Let your mother come and speak in person. I'm listening. Thus he will ask. But what word is that? A word without action, a word of disbelief. But because the man who has not studied has belief, he will say, My mother somehow will protect me. And what will the educated man say? I have education, I have money, I have everything. What do I need a god for? I have more charity than a god. Do you have the luxuries I have? Thus he will ask. But how is this? Do you understand? The educated man will suffer disease, he will suffer torment, in his family a lawsuit will arise. He will not have wisdom at all. He will have money and luxury. But he will not have the stomach to eat til his stomach is full. She will cause a disease to arise in his body. But the man who does not know how to read, look at him, if any disease comes into his body, he will say, Only you, o Mother. Gathering up sacred ash, he will put it in his mouth and say, Only you can protect me. And in the morning he will be well. He has belief. Everything will happen to the man without belief, but she will never make it better. That is her power.

When the goddess came to her in 1970, Sarasvati had reached the depths of poverty, ignominy, and despair. She was separated from her husband ("He had a religion; I had a separate religion"), had just married off her oldest daughter, and was alone with eight children to care for. "There was no food, there was no clothing, there was nothing." Her relatives shunned her because she had no money, "and with all these children, I was filthy." She and three of her daughters went to work as construction laborers, but she could not bear the painful drudgery, and she resolved one night to kill herself and all her children. That night the goddess came to her in a dream, first as a snake, then as a small child, and promised to protect her. The next day a rich woman came to Sarasvati seeking her lost husband. Speaking through Sarasvati, the goddess told her where her husband could be found, and in gratitude, the rich woman put a hundred rupees in Sarasvati's hand. After that, Sarasvati's renown spread and her wealth increased. She still maintained that the goddess would not dwell in the hearts of the rich and proud. She said that the goddess told her, "No matter how many kinsmen are yours, no matter what money they give you, your poverty will not cease .... Though you may heal many people's suffering, your own suffering will not cease." Yet she seemed to enjoy the limelight and the lovely things brought to her, and she worked hard in her profession as priestess to put as much distance as possible between her new good fortune and her past shame and poverty. She would certainly not have voluntarily returned to her previous state.

The worldly aspects of her life in some respects pleased Sarasvati, but in other respects repelled her. Living in a one-room house filled with eighteen family members, many animals and a constant stream of visitors, she often said that what she longed for most of all was peace. Sometimes, in the midst of howling babies and altercating in-laws, she would look around the room and say sadly, "There are too many people."

After Sarasvati's tenth child was born, in 1972, the goddess entered her and spoke through her to her husband, commanding him never again to touch her, or even to speak to her. She was thirty-five at the time, still of child-bearing age.

During the same year, the goddess ordered Sarasvati never again to make herself beautiful—not to comb her hair or wear ornaments of any kind. But Sarasvati disobeyed. She was ashamed when people saw her strange appearance and laughed at her. At 38 she was still a handsome woman. A photograph on the wall of the hut showed her with a fine long braid, earrings, nosering, bangles, necklaces, flowers, and silk sari—very different from the wild-looking, unadorned apparition she was now. But, Sarasvati said, now when she tried to wear earrings, the goddess would cause her ears to swell up; when she tried to wear kumkum and nose ornaments, the goddess would give her a nosebleed and headache; when she tried to comb her hair, the goddess matted it permanently overnight, angrily telling her, "I wear my form that has no comb; I wear matted hair." Thus, at the same time that Sarasvati's conjugal relations with her husband were curtailed, she was forced to give up her physical beauty.

The goddess also commanded Sarasvati not to cook or serve meals to the family, not to attend weddings or funerals, not to be attached to husband or children, to build a separate temple and live there—in effect to renounce all family and kin ties. Yet Sarasvati continued to live with her family, to love them and support them, and even, sometimes, to speak with her husband.

We do not have to delve very deeply to see that Sarasvati, growing up in an environment of changing and conflicting values, experienced mixed feelings as to her class aspirations and her role as a woman. She believed that "purity of heart" was found only in places of poverty and low status, yet she herself did not wish to be poor and despised. She believed in the value of traditional womanhood, yet she wished to be free of her family. These are just two aspects of a very complex personality, but they are significant, first, because they are problems that Sarasvati shared with a great many lower class, urban Tamil women, and second, because they enable one to understand why she became possessed by this ambivalent mother goddess, part loving and part killing, part high and part low.[12]

The characteristics of the smallpox goddess are multiple and hard to unite into a single coherent picture. She has two elemental forms, a form of wind and a form of mud. In the form of wind, bodiless spirit, she seeks a home by possessing people—"coming upon their person," in Sarasvati's idiom. In the form of mud, spiritless body, her image rises from the earth, waiting to be given life by human devotion.

The goddess loves those in whose body she dwells, except for the ones she destroys. She protects the poor and is the downfall of the rich. Thus we have learned from Sarasvati. The origin myth recounted to me by the goddess through Sarasvati tells of her once being the chaste and perfect wife of an ascetic, having magical powers of her own. Because of a trivial slip, she loses her powers, and her husband, enraged, sends her son to kill her. The son does so, decapitating both her and an untouchable woman with whom she has sought refuge. Subsequently, the son and the father repent of their rage, and the son returns to replace the mother's head upon her body. But the son bungles the job and the Brahman mother, the head, finds herself with the body of an untouchable. The husband shuns her, and she goes out into the forest to dwell alone.[13]

The goddess' name, *Māri*, means not only "rain," but also "changed," so that Māriamman is "the changed mother" as well as "the rain mother." As the rain mother, she is associated with coolness, and when she possesses her servants, she consumes great quantities of substances considered to be highly cooling: buttermilk, tumeric water, lemons, and the bitter leaves of the neem tree, whose juice heals skin diseases. Yet, though she craves cooling substances, and is called the cool one, the disease she produces is a disease of extreme heat. It used to strike during the hot, dry months, and people believe that it is caused by excess heat in the body, or by the heat of the goddess' anger. The disease is characterized by an initial high fever, and the pustules itch and burn.[14]

Consecrated to Māriamman is the month of Āḍi, the dry period of July-August, when festivals are held in her honor. But Āḍi is regarded as an in-auspicious month, when nothing new should be started: no new houses are built, and young couples live separately during that month in order to avoid conception. In general it is said that Māriamman hates the sight of a pregnant woman, and hates the sight of a married couple.[15] Some people also say that she hates children, others that she loves them.

Māriamman as the smallpox goddess may be only a few centuries old. There is evidence that *variola major*, the most virulent form of smallpox, entered India in the seventh century, but only became widely associated with a goddess

(Śītalā in Northern India) in the 16th century (see Nicholas 1981). However, the ambivalent mother goddess, possessing a shamaness and transforming her into a being at once fearsome and beautiful, is at least two millenia old, for there is a description of just such a shamaness, oracle of Kāli, in the ancient Tamil epic *Shilappadikāram*, and the bivalent goddess is a figure who appears in classical and folk texts of India throughout the ages. Therefore, the question that was posed earlier in this essay—why would a disease such as smallpox be represented as a mother?—must be turned around, and instead we must ask, why would the mother take the form of this disease? These are two rather different questions, for the former supposes that the disease itself, the physical phenomenon, determined the nature of the deity and people's response to it, whereas the latter allows us to surmise that the disease, for all its ferocity, in its religious aspect may have been only a symbol for some reality pre-dating and more fundamental to people's lives than the disease itself. Hence we may ask, if this is so, what was it about the disease that caused it to be chosen as a symbol, and what was it that it stood for?

Fortunately, we have a number of excellent monographs on the topic of smallpox, including one on the history of this disease in twentieth century Madras city by A. Ramachandra Rao, who was Medical Superintendent at the Infectious Diseases Hospital in Madras during the 1950's, 60's and 70's. These studies include in their discussions observable characteristics of the disease, or characteristics that have observable consequences, not only to specialists, but to other watchful individuals within the infected population. Herein lies the value of such studies to us, for they tell us what Madras inhabitants could themselves have noticed about smallpox—its seasons, its symptoms, who contracted it, who died of it.[16] Here are some significant details.

Smallpox is transmitted from human host to human host with no intermediate carrier; the virus is unable to survive outside of the human body for any long period of time. There is also no long latency period; within a month of infection, the host either dies of the disease or recovers and is immune (see Dixon 1962; Henderson 1976). A single infection with smallpox confers lifelong immunity; second infections are extremely rare. Sub-clinical infection (i.e., infection resulting in immunity but no noticeable symptoms) does exist, but its prevalence cannot be determined. There is some indication that the virus outside the body (in floor dirt, clothing, etc.) is less virulent; frequent contact with it may confer a high degree of immunity without causing disease.[17]

The cultural significance of these facts lies in their epidemiological consequences. Smallpox relies upon numbers for its survival, communities of several thousand persons or more, where the disease can be transmitted continuously from person to person without exhausting (either killing or rendering immune) the entire available population. Cities, and communities in contact with them, provide such an environment (see Dixon 1962; Henderson 1976). Among afflicted populations, diseases like smallpox are mainly childhood diseases. In Madras, by far the highest number of cases (59% of 3500 cases studied) occurred in children aged 0-4; the next highest number (20%) occurred in children aged 5-9. The second highest case fatality rate was among children aged 0-4 (the highest CFR was among pregnant women, for reasons to be discussed; see Rao 1972:39).

When invading a population without previous exposure, diseases like smallpox are likely to kill a high proportion of those who fall ill. Historically, the most severe smallpox epidemics have occurred among previously isolated populations upon their first intensive contact with urban populations (Dixon 1962: 189).

Among already exposed urban populations, the most severe epidemics tend to occur among sub-populations which are more isolated spatially and have less day-to-day contact with outside individuals. In India, wealthy and high-caste groups who have no contact with the dirty clothes or bodily effluvia of other groups and who live in closed compounds may be among the most vulnerable, because they have the least opportunity to gradually establish immunity to the disease. Hence a 1958 study conducted in Madras revealed that the intrafamilial transmission rate of smallpox was considerably less among the overcrowded urban poor than among the bungalow-dwelling urban rich.[18] Among the former group, the intrafamilial transmission rate of smallpox was 16 times higher than the extrafamilial transmission rate (Rao 1972: 94).

Another study, also conducted in 1958, lent further credence to the hypothesis that low-status, frequently exposed groups were at an immunological advantage with respect to smallpox. It was found in that year that an outbreak of smallpox among a community of Gounders in a village near Madras did not spread to the community of Harijans living adjacent to the Gounders in the same village. The Gounders were stoneworkers; the Harijans were agricultural laborers and scavengers (Rao 1972: 117-118).

Two main types of *variola major* were observed in Madras, hemorrhaegic and non-hemorrhaegic. The hemorrhaegic type was fatal in nearly all cases. The non-hemorrhaegic type appeared in three forms, all less severe than the hemorrhaegic type. The hemorrhaegic type was unique, also, in that it occurred with far greater frequency (80%-88%) among adults than among children; and with greatest frequency among pregnant women. Vaccination offered no protection against this type of smallpox, hence it must have been relatively more prevalent after the vaccination program started.[19]

For all types of smallpox, the case fatality rate was higher among women of childbearing age than among men; and for pregnant women the CFR was 3-4 times higher than for non-pregnant women and men. There was also a very high rate of fetal loss among women who contracted smallpox during pregnancy, 75% of cases in which smallpox was contracted in early pregnancy, and 60% of cases in which it was contracted in late pregnancy, resulted in early termination. Of children born alive to mothers who had contracted smallpox during pregnancy, 55% died within two weeks (Rao 1972: 8). Smallpox is much worse than other acute febrile diseases in this respect.

In short, in mid-twentieth century Madras city, the disease smallpox differentiated between individuals and communities according to several parameters, and it happened to draw its lines between just those categories over which Sarasvati and others like her experienced most severe conflict. Furthermore, just as these conflicts would have been felt most intensely in a cosmopolitan enivronment, the disease made its home there. It must indeed have appeared that the goddess distinguished between the rich and the poor, favoring the poor, and favoring, perhaps, most of all, members of untouchable groups, who are untouchable largely because of their contact with "dirty" things from many quarters.

It must also have seemed that the goddess favored lone individuals and did not like families, for it was within families that the disease she carried spread most readily; and she destroyed pregnancies and pregnant women with a relentlessness that must indeed have seemed horrible. With respect to children, her will was less clear: she visited them and consumed them most often, yet she saved her most severe form for adults.

The disease smallpox, then, appears to have been a ready symbol for the expression of certain aspects of the goddess, the very aspects which pulled Sarasvati away from her family and down from her aspirations for wealth and status. Yet the goddess had other aspects also.

Like shamanistic healers throughout the world, many such healers in South Asia are tested by a severe illness by means of which the deity initiates them into their new role. It seems likely that mediums of the smallpox goddess previously entered this profession through an experience of illness-cum-possession by the goddess, especially since any case of smallpox is regarded as the spirit of the mother entering the body of the afflicted individual, and since people who are ill with smallpox are believed to have oracular powers. Now, however, this process of creation and legitimization of shamanic powers vis-a-vis Māriamman can no longer take place. We return, then, to the final question posed at the beginning of this essay: what will happen (or is happening) to the cult of the smallpox goddess in Madras now that smallpox is no longer endemic there?

One answer, out of many possible ones, emerges from the experience of Sarasvati, the priestess whose life history was sketched earlier. For Sarasvati underwent a classic trial-by-illness at the hands of the smallpox goddess, but she did not contract smallpox. In a separate interview, she described this ordeal to me, and her description is worth repeating verbatim here, for it is highly illuminating.

> I was very sick. At that time this girl had been born and was seven months in the arms. At night a fever came to me. As soon as the fever came, from my belly to my chest there was a great burning. I could not eat hot spices; I could not bathe in warm water; sleep would not come; hunger would not come; if I cried "hhah," a bunch of blood would come. From my mouth I would bring up bloody bloody vomit. Then for that child, we went to see a doctor. The doctor said, This is a disease called T.B., therefore, you must be very careful. This is a very dangerous disease. In your heart, there is no power at all. It is all burned up. Therefore, you must not wear silk, you must not eat hot spices, you must drink milk with

ice in it. We must take x-rays of you. So he said. Then I said, I have children, and an unable body. When the neighbors see the disease that we have, they will be afraid. They will say, She has some kind of dangerous disease. If we go and have spoken words with her, it may come to us or something. And they will be frightened. At such a time, one cannot even bring a relative and keep them in that place. And I have to clean the children. I have to see to their food. And I have to see to my body. How can I do this? There is not even a man in the house.

At that time my father was not in Madras. My husband was a driver. The owner of the car had taken him and gone on a two month tour.

So from the doctor's office I called the owner and said, My body is very unable, it is serious, you must send the man of our house (my husband) right away. Then he said, What is the matter with your body? Then I said, I have a great bloody vomiting; the doctor said it is very serious; he is going to take me to Royapettah Hospital for x-rays, and then send me to Tambaram Hospital and commence treatment there.

As soon as I said that, what did this man do but make a long distance phone call. From the office to the house he made a long distance call. There is much danger in your house, he said. You must start home at this time. You must send your driver.

By the time he came home, my health was completely gone. It was very serious. When I lay down, at one time my whole body would be like ice, and at another time it would be boiling. I was vomiting and vomiting, and there were pearls and pearls of sweat, my whole face had darkened, my whole body had become black. I could not speak at all. If I tried to speak, there would be pain in my chest. I could only show things with my hands. That much power had been lost. Immediately, they took me to Royapettah Hospital to show me to the doctor. At that time, that mother had been in my person for only a year. We were not accustomed to being thus without the use of this body. She was in my person. But no one came to me to ask anything of her. If there had been older people, they might have done it. But there were no older people there. How could I do it myself?

It had been a year since she had come. Before the next year was over, this was a test of me. She created this disease in me to make me believe, as a way of saying, "I am here."

Out of all the doctors in Madras, one lady doctor saw me. She was called Kanaka Valli Nilāvati. That doctor too said that this was T.B. After taking the x-rays, this T.B. disease has to be treated in Tambaram. The doctor wrote a recommendation, a letter, and gave it to us. We took it, and went straight to see the doctor. She tested my whole body and said, only if you come into a dark room and let us take x-rays can we make a decision.

It was she who reminded me, the doctor who reminded me. She said, If your god is a good god, you say that you have six children, that god will protect you. You should pray that you should not have this disease. As she was taking the x-rays, she said those words to me. After she said this; she said, It would be very difficult for you to be admitted again. There are twenty injections for this. You must take these twenty injections. You must take four of these pills a day. And you must take eight of these pills a day. After that, if it is healed through that medicine, you will not need to be admitted. You must rest. You must not speak. You must not cook for anyone over fire. You rest. Otherwise, go to a peaceful temple and sit down. Or else, go to a beach and sit down by yourself. That beach wind should blow upon your person.

That day I had come wearing a silk sari. She said, Mother, you must not wear this sari. Wear an ordinary voile sari; silk is too hot. Therefore, don't you wear this. Thus she said.

After hearing all this, we came from there. As soon as we entered the house, it got worse for me. She prescribed an injection. We were wondering which doctor to go to get the injection. Then my uncle telephoned my husband at work, and he came. As soon as he came, he said I was going to go, I was going to die. My husband wrote letters to all my relatives, telling them to come. The house was full of people waiting They put me on a cot, and they turned on the fan, and kept guard. They did not have the heart to carry me away. They thought if they took me to the hospital, I would die. Besides, if we went to another hospital, how could so many people stay there and keep watch? They were expecting all of these things. Then my uncle came directly. My husband's employer gave his car and said,

If you want to take her to a doctor's house, take this car and use it. First take care of her body, she has six children; that child is a good-hearted girl, you protect her however you can. So saying, he himself, our employer, gave us five hundred rupees, and said, You must take her first to a doctor; I will recommend you to a good doctor. Whatever doctor you go and see, you telephone that doctor's address to me, I will recommend you. So that employer spoke.

After that, each day we were suffering a great agony continually. My uncle came, and took me to the doctor at Lodhra Hospital. He was a good Murugan devotee, with sacred ash on his forehead. They took me in a taxi and made me lie down in a room. The man in Lodhra Hospital looked at me and said, What does she have? They answered, This bloody vomiting will not stop, sir.

We saw doctors in all different places, and he took me to Royapettah Hospital, and gave me an injection in a vein. As soon as they gave it, it was lost. Half the needle stuck in my vein, and half the needle was broken. It stopped at the vein. It would not go in. Immediately they came there and tied ropes and things, and gave me intoxication (anesthetized me), and pushed and pulled this and that, and cut the needle and got it out.

From then on, I did not go. If they gave me an injection, it would not go into the vein. If any doctor put medicine in the needle, the medicine would not go inside. The medicine would come out. They were baffled by this. They were frightened and said that my circulation had stopped, therefore the injection would not go in. Thus they said.

With that, we left. They took me to Lodhra and made me lie down and did tests on me. He came and looked. My husband began to cry, I have this many children, it has become this serious; you must protect her, you must protect her. So saying, he wept.

Then the doctor who had comforted me said, This is nothing dangerous; whatever disease this is, I will give something for it; give her that medicine, the tonic and the pills; put a little ice cream in milk, and give it to her ice cold. If you give her that, it will be a little restful for her. Even though I haven't given her a pill to sleep, I am worried. There is much weakness in her body. You must not put any shocking news in her ear. Even if she gets better, for many days she will not have the power to bear shocks. Therefore, the god must protect her. This doctor thus spoke in the same way. Then he prescribed injections and pills and said, You must take an injection every other day. Take this pill continuously, he said.

I said, Okay. Then he said, Bring the medicine for the injection and come, not today but tomorrow. He prescribed only the injection. But when I went that day, he said, We have no injection medicine; we are out of stock; come tomorrow and take this, just take this pill, he said and gave it to me.

We came from there. When we reached the house at seven fifteen that night, they carried me to a cot and laid me down on it, and everybody, my mother and father and brothers and all had come and were sitting down crying. The children were all on one side, everybody on one side. Because of being brought in the car and the bus, I had become very tired, I was in a swoon and not aware of anything. My health was completely gone. Then laying me on that cot, everybody wept. So many people were on the doorstep wailing, O Sarasu, you good heart, you are gone, ayō, little girl, you have left all your children. In the middle of the road they were standing, really wailing and crying. I was not aware of anything.

After that, after the crying and so forth was finished, it must have been about ten-thirty, at that time a mother, well decked out, wearing a yellow sari and a yellow jacket, wearing sacred ash and kumkum, in her hand a lemon, carrying sacred ash, carrying neem leaves in one hand, an aged woman, her hair all gone white, of a ripe old age, with a bag under her arm, a bag that looked like a bag of medicine under her arm, taking that lemon and the neem leaves and sacred ash, told everyone to stand out of the way.

Except for what this old lady did, which it seemed that I saw directly and well, the weeping and all did not reach my ears.

Why, why do you cry, she said. Get out of the way. Look at this, I am going to make her well. Why do you care for her with a doctor and with medicine? Thus that mother asked.

Then from my head to my chest, that mother rubbed sacred ash and neem leaves, and said. Do you expect her life to be destroyed? This life will not be destroyed now. Only at the age of sixty-two will this life, this soul, come to peace. To make the world believe, I caused this disease to arise in this body. Even she has no belief. Therefore, to make her believe, I have caused this disease to arise. Only we can make it well. Medicine, pills, injections, you must give none of these. So speaking, she took from her bag a piece of turmeric and a green leaf. She crushed it well, and put it in a conch shell, squeezed the lemon and put the ash there, and said, you must eat only this medicine. By tomorrow, I will make a way for you to eat good food. Do you know who I am? My name is Rēnukā Paramēswari. Thus that mother said. My name is Rēnukā Paramēswari. Tomorrow I myself will come and bring about anything that you wish to happen. From this day, you must not use a doctor or take medicine. So saying, that mother disappeared.

That was all. After that, after one hour, in my health, in my body, I let out a deep breath. When I let out the breath, sweat poured from my body. I had died, they thought, and they wept. My breath had come, and without my knowing, water had come on my body. After that, I blinked my eyes, and opened them, and looked around. It was after eleven o'clock when I opened my eyes. Then everybody stopped their crying and said, There is nothing wrong with Sarasu, Sarasu has survived, she has survived, there is nothing at all wrong with her, she has nothing at all, nothing at all.

When it was still very dangerous, that mother came into my person and said, Hey, why do you have to plant a needle in her body? All the needles that you give will break. Just watch. It has been exactly a year since I have come, and you have not worshipped me. Don't come to me and ask, "Why didn't you protect her?" To make her believe, I have caused this disease to arise. From now on, blood and so forth, nothing like that will come. She will have no disease at all. Tomorrow, go take her and show her to people.

That was all. From that day to this, so far we have not given even ten rupees to a doctor. That disease does not exist in me. Otherwise, when this hot season came, this bloody vomit would always come to me. When I was pregnant I would vomit like that. Ordinarily, when the heat was excessive, it would come like this. After that mother came, she made that disease cease to exist, for eight years.

After the disease left, in the end this girl was born, and she told me in a dream. This is the seventh child, and she was born in the eighth month.

(That mother said), That seventh daughter of yours has been born. She will be in my form. You must give her my name. Call her Rēnukā Paramēswari. So she came and said.

In that way, I have called her Rēnukā Paramēswari. We had given her the name, "Love". She didn't cry, she didn't drink milk, it was as though she were dead.

That mother said, Call her by my name; I will make her cry. I will give her all powers.

After we called her Rēnukā Paramēswari, she drank milk. Today she is well. In her studies, in everything she gets the first mark. Since she was born, many astonishing things have happened in my house...

Thus the goddess tested Sarasvati, using not smallpox but tuberculosis to do so. Despite the change in disease, however, many of the key symbolic properties of smallpox remained, in new guise. For instance, one of the outstanding characteristics of smallpox, as interpreted by South Asian culture, is that it was a disease involving extremes of hot and cold. Here, Sarasvati interprets tuberculosis, which does cause chills and fever, in the same way. She said that she had a great fever, all the "power in (her) heart" (itself a significant image) was "burned up," and the doctors therefore advised her to keep her body cool and to eat milk with ice and ice cream. Instead of "pearls" of pox covering her body, there were "pearls" of sweat, and beneath the pearls, a darkened (flushed) body, such as appears with smallpox also. Bloody vomiting, too, is a symptom of smallpox.

More importantly, for Sarasvati this illness experience was associated with pregnancy and childbirth. At the time the illness climaxed, she had one seven-month-old baby in the arms and was pregnant with another. The child that was subsequently born nearly died, but was saved, like Sarasvati, by the intervention of the goddess. This baby was the seventh child and the sixth daughter. Six daughters were a great burden for Sarasvati, because of the necessity of marrying them all off, with dowries and expensive festivities. But the goddess transformed this last daughter into a blessing, investing her with great intellectual and magical powers.

Sarasvati's illness experience was also associated with the break-up of the family and absence of family support. Her husband was out of town and her relatives would not speak to her because she had a contagious disease. On the bed of her near death and miraculous revival, she was united with her kin, yet as we have seen earlier, the goddess' will was that this reunion not be permanent.

Also striking is the way that, in Sarasvati's dreaming and remembering, the goddess and the woman doctor sometimes merged, sometimes clashed. Though the goddess came in the form of a doctor, with a medicine bag under her arm, she broke all the needles that were forced into Sarasvati's body, and finally commanded Sarasvati never to visit a doctor or use medicine again. Sarasvati was to be independent, separate and non-cosmopolitan, and her body was to be no one's domain but the goddess'. The doctor for her part was sympathetic to Sarasvati's faith, and reinforced the hot-cold interpretation of her sickness. The advice she gave Sarasvati was remarkably similar to the commands the goddess herself had issued: remove yourself from others, don't cook, don't speak, don't wear fancy, heavy clothing, let the cool beach wind blow (like a possessing spirit) upon your person. Recovery from tuberculosis required, as Sarasvati remembers it, the same renunciation of family life that devotion to the goddess entailed.

Why did the goddess employ tuberculosis to test Sarasvati? Was there anything about this disease that made it, like smallpox, an apt vehicle of the goddess' message ?

Tuberculosis in Madras is far more common than smallpox ever was; indeed, it is the most destructive disease in the city. In 1958, the tuberculosis morbidity rate there was estimated at 2.5% .[20] In a city of about two million, fifty thousand people were ill with tuberculosis. Today, Madras may have largest stable tubercular population of any city in the world.[21] Even more than smallpox, tuberculosis is a disease associated with the process of urbanization, being transmitted from person to person and being most endemic in relatively dense populations. It is also associated with modernization; because it is a complex, slow-moving disease with varying symptoms, its recognition as a disease is historically fairly recent. There is no indigenous Tamil word for it. Hence Sarasvati uses the English term "T.B." to refer to it.

In some respects, tuberculosis is the exact opposite (a symbolic inverse) of smallpox. Smallpox comes during the hot, dry months; tuberculosis thrives in dark, damp places. Whereas infection with smallpox leads either to death or recovery and immunity within a fairly short period of time, initial infection with tuberculosis bacilli does neither. Most commonly, upon first infection, there are no visible symptoms. The bacteria multiply for a few weeks until the body develops an allergic reaction to the bacilli and encases them in tubercles of giant, multi-nucleated cells or in caseous material formed by dead tissue. The lesion is in effect healed and the patient well, although small numbers of bacteria remain alive, contained within the tubercle of caseous material.

However, subsequent re-infection may occur when for some reason the person's resistance is lowered and the effectiveness of the allergic response is reduced. Endogenous reinfection may occur if the tubercle is broken or caseous material liquified and the contained bacteria are liberated into the bloodstream. Or re-infection may be exogenous. In any case, whereas the primary focus of tubercular infection tends to heal, subsequent re-infection tends to remain smouldering and gradually to spread. Thus, a person may be initially infected with tuberculosis and only develop symptoms years later. And then the disease may continue for years, with the individual's conditions becoming progressively worse. Incidence of the disease is a function of chances for exposure and the degree to which the general state of health is low (Cruikshank 1965: 197-198).

The onset of symptoms frequently follows some trauma or mental or physical stress, exhaustion or malnutrition[22]—all of these conditions being very much present among the urban poor, and especially being associated with childbirth among poor women. It is perhaps for this reason that mortality statistics are higher among females of childbearing age than among males (Wolansky 1980:734; Rich 1951: 183).[23]

The onset of symptoms may also be precipitated by trauma due to the loss of loved ones or break-up of families (Jayasuriya 1967: 154-161).[24] Thus whereas smallpox destroys pregnancies, pregnant women, and families, with tuberculosis this causal relation is in a sense reversed: pregnancy and childbirth may (as in Sarasvati's case) bring about the onset of tubercular symptoms, or aggrevate these symptoms, as may the break-up of families. Whatever the actual causal sequence, however, tuberculosis and smallpox are alike in their strong association with bad pregnancies and ruined families. It may be added that tuberculosis, like smallpox (and many other diseases), takes its greatest toll among small children.

The spread of tuberculosis is facilitated by crowded and dirty living conditions and by frequent and close contact with strangers, but unlike with smallpox, these conditions do not raise the level of immunity within the exposed population. Hence the urban poor have always borne the brunt of this disease. Whereas smallpox distinguishes between the high and the low, tending to spare the low, tuberculosis makes the same distinction, but favors instead the high.

A kind of folk-etiology has arisen in conjunction with tuberculosis in India, associating it with slum-living and untouchability. It is thought by many to be hereditary, and to result from bad karma, immoral habits and bad company. An individual who has had the disease may be shunned or ostracized by neighbors and kin (as was Sarasvati), and someone who is known to have had tuberculosis, even if they have recovered, may find it very difficult to get a job or a marriage partner. Hence tuberculosis tends to draw attention to, and to aggravate, the very conditions which give rise to it: poverty, low status, physical vulnerability, and the loosening or breaking of kin ties concomitant upon migration to and settlement in the city. To admit to having tuberculosis is to emphasize one's identity as a slum-dweller, and to classify oneself together with a very large number of people whose status is low and whose lives are hard.

Sarasvati sometimes would say of the mother whom she worshipped, she dwells in many places and she has many names and many forms, but she is one deity only, and one power. Thus many Hindus speak of their chosen deities. A deity which had only one meaning could probably not reach far into many people's hearts and would probably not last long. In the case of Māriamman, it is clear that she truly is a changed and changing mother in her aspect of disease goddess and patroness of the urban poor and married women, and still there are other aspects of her that we have not even examined. Beyond being a symbol, she is herself a maker of symbols, a power flowing through changing times, forms, and conditions.

In this essay I have shown how the personality of Māriamman gives expression to some of the more severe conflicts experienced by the priestess Sarasvati and gives her the power, indeed compels her, to face these conflicts and settle them. For reasons that have been recounted, the disease smallpox seems to have served as a convenient symbol for a number of common and interrelated problems: the pain and stigma of poverty, family discord, the oppression of crowded living conditions and too many mouths to feed, the threat to women's health of multiple pregnancies. In Sarasvati's time, smallpox was no longer available as a symbol, but another disease, tuberculosis, represented equally well and perhaps better the same realities. When these realities threatened to crush Sarasvati, as they had done to many before her, the goddess entered into (or emerged from) Sarasvati's heart and enabled her to free herself, at least to some extent, from her troubled condition. Sarasvati's triumph over tuberculosis confirmed in her a certain moral identity, just as a similar bout with smallpox would have done. However the disease was not the source of this identity, nor was it the source of the goddess who aided her. The demise of a particular disease did not, in essence, effect the goddess at all. From what we have seen it seems probable that, as long as struggles such as Sarasvati's take place, whatever diseases come and go, deities like Māriamman will remain alive.

NOTES

1   It is misleading to think of Hindu deities as objects or symbols which are manipulated by human actors, because these deities operate, for the most part, in realms which are entirely beyond the control of individuals—the realms of subconscious drives and of social forces. It can be argued that one reason deities appear so powerful is that they unite into a single presence elements of both the subconscious and the social. This presence is composed of an array of symbols which speak to the human individual and compel him or her to behave in certain ways. The great flexibility of Hindu deities is a consequence of the polyvalence of the symbols composing them, and the capacity of such symbols to link in different ways with different contextual symbols to form a large number of different messages.

2   Cf., for instance, the discussion of demons and *pretas* by Obeyesekere (1981), of marital relations of dominance and subordination by Daniel (1980), and of general codes for conduct by Singer (1972).

3   Few, if any, of these characteristics of healers are confined to South Asian cultures. See for instance Hallowell (1941), Geertz (1960), Frank (1961), Kiev (1968), Lewis (1971), Crapanzano (1977)), Landy (1977).

4   Rivalry, rather than cooperation, marks the relations between the different healing traditions in Madras city. Cosmopolitan and Āyurvedic medicine and learned religious healing (cf. Leslie 1976) all are high-status, male-dominated professions whose practitioners look down upon trance-healers, even when the former recognize the reality of spirit possession. Especially lamented by these high-status professionals is the fact that so many Harijans resort to trance-healers even when more "scientific" forms of medicine are readily available. On a fundamental level, however, all of these medical traditions, including both Indian cosmopolitan medicine and trance-healing, share a common set of assumptions and are mutually complementary (Egnor 1983).

5   One of the most notable indications of the legitimation of Māriamman's authority is the employment of Brahman priests at the Tiruvērkāḍu temple. Traditionally, because the goddess demands blood sacrifice, South Indian Brahmans have avoided connection with her. At the Tiruvērkāḍu temple, she now accepts only vegetarian offerings.

6   In the Malayāli branch of Āyurveda, every disease has its own associated demon. In Madras, Māriamman herself is used to exorcise demons: her spirit calls to the possessing spirit and leads it away from the body of the afflicted person. In Sinhalese demon exorcism, the Buddha is invoked to bring disease demons under control.

7   For a detailed discussion of this association, see Egnor (1978).

8   See Nicholas 1981; Nicholas and Sarkar 1976.

9   The actual number of cases of smallpox that occurred was probably higher, perhaps much higher, than the number of cases reported, even after the W.H.O. program began. Henderson (1976) reports serious mismanagement of the smallpox eradication program in India. Searches for cases were inefficient, and in some areas, were never even conducted, and known outbreaks of smallpox were concealed. After these abuses were discovered, a new program of intensive and thorough house-to-house searches was carried out, first in a single district of southern India, and then, when this proved successful, throughout the subcontinent. Cases were isolated, and through vaccination of all those in contact with the patient, outbreaks were eliminated, region by region. Madras has been officially smallpox-free since 1970, and was certainly smallpox-free by 1973. The last case of smallpox in India, according to the W.H.O., occurred in May, 1975.

10 Māriamman was previously one of a number of "village goddesses" whose worship, though widespread, was not centralized in major temples as was the worship of the great Sanskritic deities. Village-level deities are commonly housed in small mud shrines or featureless stones, and their mythology, though not unrelated to Purāṇic and other written texts, was transmitted orally. Hence there is no way of knowing for sure how long Māriamman has been around.

11 The life history sketched here is derived entirely from Sarasvati's own account—the events of the past filtered through her memory. What is recounted, and all that is important for the

purposes of this paper, is not what "really happened" (i.e., an amalgam of various points of view) but what affected Sarasvati and what she believes happened—how she sees herself in relation to the world and in relation to the goddess. Obeyesekere (1981), in his study of a number of female ascetics similar to the one described here, adopted a similar methodology. My approach differs from his, however, in that I see this paper as essentially a translation of a message that Sarasvati herself was trying to get across to me; Obeyesekere is concerned with developing Western psychoanalytic and sociological theory on the basis of what he has learned *about* his informants, *through* their messages to him.

12   A future paper will focus upon the significance of the ambivalent mother goddess to female worshippers such as Sarasvati.

13   Whitehead (1921) found the same origin myth for Māriamman as village goddess. A variant of the same story appears in Sanskrit literature. There the name of the heroine is Rēnukā Paremēswari—the name that Sarasvati, at the goddess' command, gives to her seventh daughter.

14   Other discussions of the hot-and-cold character of the smallpox goddess in northern and southern India appear in Beck (1969) and Wadley (1980).

15   Babb (1970) reports the same belief in central India.

16   As Nicholas points out (1981: 23), it is wrong to suppose that, just because Indian people place a religious interpretation upon certain events, they are ignorant of the natural properties of those events. Detailed understanding of particular events in the natural world may in fact be accompanied by great elaboration of the *meaning* of those events, and considerable symbolic, as well as practical use of them. In Tamil Nadu, plant growth is one such factually well-understood and symbolically highly elaborated domain. Smallpox may well have been another.

17   Rao (1972: 78-79, 98-108) makes this connection. Other writers note the existence of varying degrees of immunity to smallpox, of sub-clinical infection, and of the persistence of the virus outside the body for periods of up to a year (e.g., Rhodes and van Rooyen, 1958; Rivers, 1948). The causes of sub-clinical infection, and of immunity to smallpox in individuals who have neither been vaccinated nor previously developed a frank case of the disease, have not been established. According to Rao, "Studies on intrafamilial transmission of smallpox indicated that nearly 60 percent of the unvaccinated, and as high as 98 percent of the vaccinated, escape clinical disease even on close exposure to smallpox" (p. 98). After citing much laboratory evidence, he concludes, "Not only do subclinical cases occur, but they occur far more frequently than one would expect" (p. 108). The reason for such a high incidence of sub-clinical disease in Madras may be frequent, low-level exposure to the virus conferring partial immunity, or immunity without serious illness; one possible source of low-level exposure is virus which has been outside the body for some time. Holwell (1767, cited by Nicholas, 1981) described a technique of variolation employed by specialists in Bengal in which patients were inoculated with matter from "the inoculated pustules of the previous year, for they never inoculate with fresh matter." The diminished virulence of virus long outside the body would make sense of such a practice.

Other possible reasons for high resistance to smallpox among certain groups are discussed below (note 26). Whatever the cause, Rao's epidemiological evidence suggests that resistance to smallpox within the Madras population as a whole was "comparatively high," and a higher level of resistance existed among low status groups and those living in overcrowded and dirty conditions than among others,

Interestingly, Dixon reports that in England also, in the 17th and 18th centuries prior to the introduction of variolation, smallpox was "a disease of the nobility."

18   See Rao (1972: 117). The severity of a case of smallpox, as of many other diseases, may be effected not only by the immunological status of the host, but also by the host's nutritional status, and possibly also by genetic factors.

On the subject of natural immunity to smallpox, Rivers (1948) says:

It is well known that excellent health is no protection against measles, influenza, chickenpox and smallpox, Furthermore, it is a definite impression of many people working with viruses that unhealthy animals are either more resistant or react less severely to certain viral maladies than do perfectly normal animals. Indeed, as long ago as the time of Jenner there was talk of and reports regarding certain individuals being less susceptible to vaccinia because of the presence in them of other diseases. These observations were taken to indicate that as a result of some previous or concomitant disease individuals were not so highly susceptible to other kinds of disease as they would have been had they been perfectly healthly.

Regarding nutrition, Nicholas (1981) has shown that increases in smallpox mortality in the eighteenth, nineteenth, and early twentieth centuries can be correlated with drought and famine. Since smallpox may be contracted by inhalation of virus particles, drought (unrelieved by the rain mother!) facilitates the spread of the disease by enabling the virus to travel with the wind through the dry dusty air. In any given year, the prevalence of the disease reached its peak during the dry season.

Famine increases the mortality rate from smallpox because recovery from this disease is dependent upon the host's ability to rebuild destroyed tissue in a short period of time, which ability in turn is dependent upon nutritional factors, most notably, protein consumption.

The interplay of nutritional, immunological, genetic and sociological variables in determining the epidemiology of a disease is surely subtle, and probably differs from region to region. In Bengal, the repeated occurrence of severe famines rendered the poor during these times more vulnerable to death even from lesser diseases (Sen 1981). In Madras, where famine has been far less prevalent, the nutritional differential between high-status and low-status groups is modified by the relative absence of food prohibitions among the lower status groups. Crabs, snails, rats, and larger animals form an important part of the diet of many low-caste groups, whereas high-caste groups are often vegetarian, and may have restricted access even to milk. Until quite recently, the poor in Tamil Nadu also relied upon millet (a relatively high-protein grain) as a staple, rather than rice, which was considered a luxury food. This is not to say that the poor are better nourished than the rich, but only that the nutritional profile of different social groups in Madras, especially with respect to protein consumption, is complex.

19 Rao (1972: 8) writes that in the "early hemorrhaegic" variety of smallpox, 88% of the cases reported were among adults and 66% of these were among pregnant women. In the "late hemorrhaegic" variety, 80% of cases were among adults, with pregnant woman "slightly more susceptible". For all varieties of smallpox combined, the case fatality rate was higher among women 15-44 than among men, and three to four times higher among pregnant women than among non-pregnant women and men.

20 *New York Times*, January 20, 1980.

21 *New York Times*, January 20, 1980.

22 "Epidemiological evidence on the frequency of tuberculosis has long suggested that malnutrition, overcrowding, and stress decrease resistance to the disease" (Wolansky 1980: 731; see also Rich 1951: 614-661).

23 According to Rich, in some populations the female mortality rate from tuberculosis remains higher from puberty on. It is likely that India is one such population, because of the generally higher female mortality rate at all ages there (Miller 1981). The reasons for the differential between male and female tubercular mortality rates are unestablished, but Rich, after considering in detail a number of possible reasons, provides convincing evidence that childbearing is to blame. He concludes, "... regardless of the differences of opinion that exist concerning the advisability of permitting a tuberculous woman to bear a child *if adequate care is provided before and after labor,* it is beyond question that if adequate care and rest are *not* assured (and certainly, they are not assured in the case of most tuberculous women who become pregnant), childbearing may be attended by a variety of circumstances of a nature known to affect tuberculosis adversely. It is recognized, for example, that physical exertion, malnutrition, insufficient sleep and mental strain all exert an unfavorable influence upon tuberculosis, and childbearing commonly entails one or more of these unfavorable influences (Rich 1951: 196-197; emphasis his).

24 Overcrowding is also frequently cited as a factor increasing vulnerability to tuberculosis, both because of the increased chances for exposure and because of the increased stress that it

entails (e.g. Cruikshank 1965: 199; Wolansky 1980: 731). Since overcrowding is likely to be a source of family discord as well, the three-sided association is tightened: tuberculosis both causes and is precipitated by family discord; family discord is aggravated by overcrowding; and overcrowding is involved in both the biological and emotional causation of the overt disease. Tuberculosis thus is both symptom and powerful symbol of the hardships of poverty and excessive family pressures. That treatment of the disease involves both rest and isolation makes it all the more inviting as a means of communication of these troubles, and as a temporary way out.

REFERENCES

ADIGAL, Ilango
    1965 *Shilappadikaram*. Alain Danielou, trans. New York: New Directions.
BABB, Lawrence
    1970 "Marriage and Malevolence: the Uses of Sexual Opposition in a Hindu Pantheon." *Ethnology* 9(2): 137-148.
BECK, Brenda, E. F.
    1969 "Color and Heat in South Indian Ritual." *Man* 4(4): 553-572.
CRAPANZANO, Vincent
    1977 "Introduction." *In* Vincent Crapanzano and Vivian Garrison (eds.), *Case Studies in Spirit Possession*. New York: John Wiley. Pp. 1-40.
CRUIKSHANK, Walter
    1965 *Medical Microbiology*. Baltimore: Wilkins and Williams.
DANIEL, Sherry
    1980 "Marriage in Tamil Culture. The Problem of Conflicting 'Models'." *In* Susan S. Wadley (ed.), *The Powers of Tamil Women*. Syracuse: Maxwell School of Citizenship and Public Affairs, Syracuse University.
DIXON, C. W.
    1962 *Smallpox*. London: J. and A. Churchill.
EGNOR, Margaret
    1978 The Sacred Spell and Other Conceptions of Life in Tamil Culture. Unpublished Ph.D. dissertation, Department of Anthropology, University of Chicago.
    1983 "Death and Nurturance in Indian Systems of Healing." *Social Science and Medicine* 17 (14): 935-945.
FRANK, Jerome
    1961 *Persuasion and Healing*. Baltimore: The Johns Hopkins Press.
GEERTZ, Clifford
    1960 *The Religion of Java*. New York: The Free Press.
HALLOWELL, Irving
    1941 "The Social Function of Anxiety in a Primitive Society." *American Sociological Review* 7: 869-881.
HENDERSON, Donald A.
    1976 "The Eradication of Smallpox." *Scientific American* 245 (Oct.): 25-33.
HOLWELL, J. Z.
    1767 *An Account of the Manner of Inoculating for the Smallpox in the East Indies*. London: College of Physicians. (Reprinted in Dharampal, *Indian Science and Technology in the Eighteenth Century: Some Contemporary European Accounts*. Delhi: Impex India. 1971).
JAYASURIYA, J. H. F.
    1967 *The Challenge of Tuberculosis*. Columbo, Sri Lanka: The Wesley Press.
KIEV, Ari.
    1968 *Curanderismo: Mexican-American Folk Psychiatry*. New York: The Free Press.
LANDY, David
    1977 "Conceptions of Healing Statuses and Roles." *In* David Landy (ed.), *Culture, Disease, and Healing*. New York: Macmillan.

LESLIE, Charles
    1976   "The Ambiguities of Medical Revivalism in Modern India." *In* Charles Leslie
        (ed.), *Asian Medical Systems*. Berkeley: University of California Press. Pp. 356-367.
LEWIS, I. M.
    1971   *Ecstatic Religion*. Middlesex: Penguin Books.
MILLER, Barbara
    1981   *The Endangered Sex: Neglect of Female Children in Rural North India*. Ithaca: Cornell
        University Press.
NICHOLAS, Ralph
    1981   "The Goddess Sitala and Epidemic Smallpox in Bengal." *Journal of Asian Studies*
        41(1): 21-44.
NICHOLAS, Ralph and Aditi Nath SARKAR
    1976   "The Fever Demon and the Census Commissioner: Sitala Mythology in Eighteenth
        and Nineteenth Century Bengal." *In* Marvin Davis (ed.), *Bengal: Studies in Literature,*
        Society, and History. East Lansing: Michigan State University, Asian Studies Center
        Occasional Papers (South Asia Series No. 27). Pp. 3-68.
OBEYESEKERE, Gananath.
    1981   *Medusa's Hair*. Chicago: University of Chicago Press.
RAO, A. Ramachandra.
    1972   *Smallpox*. Bombay: Kothari Book Depot.
RHODES, Andrew J. and E. E. VAN ROOYEN
    1958   *A Textbook of Virology*. 3d edition. Baltimore: Wilkins and Williams.
RICH, Arnold R.
    1951   *The Pathogenesis of Tuberculosis*. 2d edition. Springfield, Illinois: Charles C. Thomas.
RIVERS, Thomas M.
    1948   *Viral and Rickettsial Infections of Man*. New York J. B. Lippincott Co.
SEN, Amartya
    1981   Poverty and Famine: An Essay on Environment and Deprivation. London: Oxford
        University Press.
SINGER, Milton
    1972   "Industrial Leadership, the Hindu Ethic, and the Spirit of Socialism." *In* Milton
        Singer, *When a Great Tradition Modernizes*. New York: Praeger.
WADLEY, Susan S.
    1980   "Sitala: The Cool One." *Asian Folklore Studies* 39(1): 33-62.
WHITEHEAD, Henry
    1921   *Village Gods of South India*. London: Oxford University Press.
WOLANSKY, Emanuel
    1980   "Microbacteria" *In* Bernhard D. Davis, Renato Dulbaco, Harman N. Eisen, and
        Harold S. Ginsberg, *Microbiology*. 3d edition. New York: Harper and Row.

Time and the Process of Diagnosis in Sinhalese Ritual Treatment*

LORNA AMARASINGHAM RHODES

University of Maryland, Baltimore, U.S.A.

RECENTLY THE NOTION OF DIAGNOSIS as a simple process of naming—the equivalent of "appending names to trees" (Good 1977)—has been called into question in a number of related fields. The diagnostic process is coming to be seen as just that, a process, involving complex relationships among social, cultural and historical factors. The influence of the patient's social network on diagnostic decisions (e.g. Waxler 1977; Zola 1973), the effect of historical contexts on popular diagnoses of the past (e.g. neurasthenia [Sicherman 1977] and masturbation [Engelhardt 1974]), and the existence of diagnoses unrecognized by Western medicine (e.g. Good 1977; Obeyesekere 1976), all suggest the extent to which diagnosis, like treatment itself, must be understood as a complex symbolic undertaking.

In studies of ritual the diagnostic aspect of treatment often gets lost in the intricacy of the ritual process; especially when the diagnostician is someone other than the ritual specialist, as in cases where diviners make the initial diagnosis, it is easy for diagnosis to be seen as simple naming even when ritual is described in all its symbolic complexity. In this paper I will look at a case of ritual treatment in which diagnosis stands out as a central issue. The problematic relationship between diagnosis and cure in the case presented here illustrates: (1) how symptoms take on weight and meaning in a dynamic interaction with symbolic aspects of treatment, and (2) how this action unfolds paradoxically and non-lineally through time.

The most general question addressed here is: How does a diagnosis develop over time? I present the case of a Sinhalese woman in Sri Lanka treated for barrenness attributed to the influence of a demon (*yaka*), a malevolent supernatural of the Sinhalese pantheon.[1] By looking at the process of attribution—at how the patient becomes "a woman afflicted with a demon"—we see how the patient's condition comes to be perceived as embodying the meanings associated with a particular demon. Two more specific questions are contained within this larger one. One is: What is the relationship

* *Acknowledgments.* I would like to thank T. Abeyrama for his assistance in Sri Lanka, and E. V. Daniel, G. Obeyesekere, and H. L. Seneviratne for their comments on an earlier version of this paper.

between *time* and *diagnosis* in this case? Since it unfolds in time in an unusual way (though in a way not atypical for the Sinhalese) it suggests the artificiality of separating the curative from the diagnostic aspects of treatment, and further, points to the complex ways in which ritual and diagnosis can be temporally related. The other question relates to a previous paper in which I show how a Sinhalese patient and her family move from healer to healer in search of a cure for madness (Amarasingham 1980). In that case the patient and family sought out a variety of diagnoses for the illness which then coexisted in a very fluid network of explanation. If such fluidity is, as I think it is, common, then the case discussed here raises a complementary question: What does make a diagnosis 'stick'? If instead of assuming that most diagnoses have a one-to-one relation to an illness we assume that they can often be conditional or not fully descriptive of the patient's condition, then what contributes to the permanence and stability of those diagnoses which are recognized as final?

This case, like the previous one, is based on retrospective material and therefore is constructed from the commentary of the ritualist, the patient, and her family. This method, while it does not provide enough detail on how decisions about treatment are actually made, has the advantage of clearly revealing the "weight" of various diagnoses in the final analysis made by the participants. While the family described in the previous paper went into detail about all the treatments sought, in this family, where one diagnosis became dominant, other treatments were given only the most cursory attention.

The ritual described here was observed during field work in 1977 in the Kotmale area of Sri Lanka, a mountainous region near Kandy where the Sinhalese people live in small agricultural villages. My assistant and I talked at length with the *Kaṭṭaḍiyā* (ritual exorcist, here called G.) before and after he performed the ritual described here. We visited the patient's (here called P.M.) home twice after the ritual and talked with her and several members of her family. I was already familiar with the ritual and the practitioner as a result of earlier field work in the area.

The supernatural explanation for affliction which is central to this case is one of many in Sinhalese thought about illness. Demons (*yakās*) are malevolent beings who are low in the hierarchy of the supernatural pantheon and who attack humans, particularly those who are vulnerable in certain ways. Ritual cures for demonically caused illness are based on two assumptions rooted in the Sinhalese religious system as a whole: (1) That demons are subject to the higher authority of the gods who are above them and that they must therefore obey gods who are invoked and enlisted on the side of the ritual practitioner, and (2) that demons accept food and other offerings as compensation for "giving up" a human victim. In other words, it is assumed that one can successfully negotiate with supernatural beings. Rituals to placate demons are elaborate, colorful, and expensive. They are usually performed by a troupe of specialists consisting of a chief exorcist, drummers, dancers, and assistants. Smaller rituals (such as the vow which is important in the case to follow) are performed only by the exorcist and are usually quite short, simple, and inexpensive.

Western medicine, which also figures in this case, is widely available and virtually free.

The Case History

When my assistant and I met the patient, P.M., she was twenty-nine years old and had given birth to her first child three months earlier. She was living in her mother's house while she and her husband completed a new house on some newly acquired land. The family was poor and lived in the less desirable area of the village near the lower reaches of a tea plantation. P.M. was the sixth of eleven brothers and sisters. No one in the family had more than a fourth grade education, and the older brothers worked as day laborers on the tea estate while rotating tenure of the 3/4 acre plot belonging to the mother. The father, who had cultivated this plot, had been dead about five years.

When P. M. was in her early teens a relative died in her house. She was asked to go to tell her married sister who lived several miles away. She had to walk the distance, and while she was walking her first menstruation began. When she arrived at her sister's house the ritual for first menstruation (*kotahalu*)[2] was immediately begun and carried to completion without incident. An important component of this ritual is the protection of the girl from malign supernatural influences. However, the Sinhalese believe that to be alone (*tanikama*) during one's first menstruation and also to be in contact with death are factors which make one vulnerable to demonic attack. P.M. said, nevertheless, that once the ritual had been performed she did not worry about the possible efects of this incident.

In 1968 P.M. was married to a young man from a nearby village; he was a relative of hers and her parents approved the match (see Yalman 1967 on Kandyan kinship). During the period from 1968 to 1976 she had five miscarriages (most around the third of fourth month) and was unable to carry a pregnancy to term. P.M. and her family were somewhat vague in talking about their initial reactions to the problem. At one point they said that after the first miscarriage they went to a fortuneteller who diagnosed *Kadavara doṣa* (trouble caused by the demon Kadavara), and that because the illness was known to be caused by Kadavara, P.M. was not blamed for it by her husband or his family. At another point, however, they said that they only realized much later that a ritual for Kadavara was necessary. During her years of barrenness P.M. went to many temples, went on pilgrimages, and had a number of minor rituals performed. After each miscarriage, she went to the local medical clinic for treatment, but she did not consult the medical practitioner about how to prevent future miscarriages.

Either just before or very shortly after the beginning of her most recent pregnancy P.M.'s family went to G.[3] They described her situation and he recommended a ritual for the Kadavara demon to be performed after the taking of a vow (*bhara*). Vows are common in Sinhalese life and involve the promise to a god or demon that if an illness or misfortune ends, certain offerings or sacrifices will be made. One advantage to the person making the vow is that it is small and inexpensive, whereas the larger ritual which is promised is quite expensive; for example, the cost of a ritual might be equivalent to a month of a day laborer's pay. P.M. had already made a number of vows, but none to Kadavara or any other demons.

G. performed the vow at P.M.'s house shortly after the family's visit to him.[4] To make the vow, a new pot is filled with an egg, jaggery, paddy, and a coconut. This is tied with an areca-nut leaf and on the outside a simple *yantra* (magical diagram) is drawn with lime. An invocation is then made to the gods, particularly the Kohomba god who is, according to G., Kadavara's immediate superior. The invocations promise Kadavara a ritual (the *Kadavara Pidīma*, an offering to Kadavara) to be performed between the third and seventh month of the child's life. The pot is then hung over the patient's bed, where it remains throughout the pregnancy.

In the fourth month of her pregnancy, P.M. went to the local medical clinic, where she was referred to the hospital in a neighboring town. She remained at the hospital for eighteen days and received injections for high blood pressure.[5] She returned to the hospital again in the eighth month for further treatment. A few weeks before the child was born she returned to the hospital, where she was delivered by Caesarean section. P.M. stressed that she felt it was the vow, not the medical treatment, which had made the birth possible. Her mother added emphatically "What can doctors know about this?"

The ritual in fulfillment of the vow had been planned for the beginning of the third month after the birth. But because of another ritual which had been scheduled in the family, P.M. and her husband changed the date to the seventh day of the third month. During the seven days of waiting for the performance P.M. said that the baby became very restless and "was afraid of his dreams." He could not be comforted, and this confirmed her belief that without the ritual Kadavara would make the child ill or perhaps even kill it.

The family members pointed out to us several times the protective aspects of the vow and ritual. The demons, they said, were prevented from coming into the house by the ritual of the vow; they were waiting to get in and thus it was important to perform the full exorcism ritual inside even though the house was small and poor. P.M. felt that this ritual would be effective for future pregnancies and that she no longer needs to worry about whether she can bear children, though she expects future children also to be delivered by Caesarean.

The Development of the Diagnosis

The diagram shows how the patient's history relates to the diagnostic process. At first the possibility of demonic affliction exists because of the events surrounding P.M.'s first menstruation, but it is not given concrete form. Then, as she miscarries repeatedly, a number of diagnostic trials are undertaken, such as pilgrimages and vows at temples. These, when unsuccessful, are almost forgotten. The family's vagueness about when the Kadavara diagnosis

emerged as central reflects the fact that Kadavara was one of a gradually nar-
rowing field of possibilities.

The family describes, then, a movement from diffuse suspicion to the cer-
tainty of a specific demon as cause of the illness. This movement, as they suggest when they mention that P.M. is not to blame for her barrenness, probably
corresponds to a lessening of guilty and painful immersion in the barrenness
through an interpretation which provides symbolic distance from private
aspects of the illness (cf. Amarasingham 1980). When they describe the vow as
protective of P.M., they are describing the power of the ritual hanging of the
pot to distance the demon from her, creating a magical barrier to its intrusion
into her body by shifting the demon's attention to the boundary (*sima*) created
around the house.

The time-line illustrates how, in this case, one diagnosis comes into focus
and has meaning and permanence for the patient and all the members of her
family. Although other kinds of healing are involved (Western medicine,
pilgrimages, etc.), none takes on a similar centrality. Obviously one reason for
this is that the patient carried her pregnancy to term after taking the vow. If she
had not, Kadavara probably would have gone the way of the other tentative interpretations. However, the (to our minds) obvious importance of Western
medicine was dismissed by P.M. and her family in favor of what was clearly
the more compelling explanation. I will turn now to some of the other factors
which contribute to the strength of the explanation based on Kadavara.

The Relationship between Women's Reproductive Role and Demonic Affliction

The Sinhalese believe that demons are attracted to certain areas of
vulnerability in human life. For example, they attack at transitional times of
day and are attracted to "aloneness" (*tanikama*, also a synonym for demonically caused illness), whether physical or psychological. Through menstruation
and childbirth women are closer to the processes of life and death than men,
and these processes involve substances (blood and other body fluids) which are
particularly attractive to demons. Demons can be important to women quite
apart from their reproductive function and can become a means through which
women express aggression or sexuality (Obeyesekere 1977; Kapferer 1974).
Women can also use possession trance to express an individual relationship to
a specific demon (Obeyesekere 1977). The demonic influence on menstruation, sexuality and childbirth, however, affects all women. The puberty ritual,
for instance, is explicit about the danger to women from demonic attack.

Because of this notion of general susceptibility the presence of demons is
important in the daily life of Sinhalese women. It is a link between private experience and public expectation. Women cannot be alone, go out alone
(especially at night), or engage in certain activities because this makes them
vulnerable to demons. The restrictions on girls' activities which begin at
puberty are phrased in terms of demonic danger as well as in social terms.

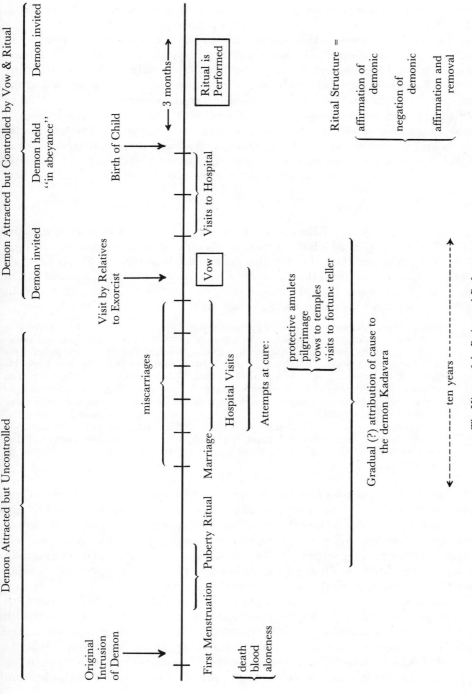

The History of the Patient and Performance

Thus, demons constitute one phrasing of the rules governing female sexuality, which must be guarded if it is to function properly.

I do not have enough information on P.M. to say whether she made connections between elements in her inner life (say, the relationship to a male figure, as in Obeyesekere's case) and the "personality" of her afflicting demon. She seemed free of psychological symptoms and I would guess that she did not. Nevertheless, she had a relationship to the demon which unfolded in her life around her reproductive condition, and this kind of relationship, I think, is more common for Sinhalese women than the more complex one of psychological identification. The diagnosis of *Kadavara doṣa*, then, derives some of its strength from an identification between women and demons which exists as a potential tension around the reproductive life of women.

The Kadavara Demon

The ritual offering of Kadavara is related to a major Kandyan ritual, the *Kohoṁba Kaṅkāriya*, in which the demon Kadavara is one member of the retinue of the Kohomba god (one of the twelve gods of the Kandyan area). Kadavara's connection to the mythical themes of the *Kaṅkāriya* is probably less important in this context, however, than the origin story associated with him. This story is associated with Kadavara in the Kotmale area:

> A king had two children. Fortunetellers predicted that they would commit incest so the king took the sister away and hid her. When the boy grew up he heard about his sister and asked everyone where she was, but no one would tell him. When the sister reached puberty the *dhobi* (washerwoman) who attended the *Kotahalu* ritual met the boy on her way back. He threatened her and finally she told him about his sister. He went to the king and insisted on seeing her. When they brought the sister in to see him they put a curtain between them so that they could only see one another's faces. Even so as soon as the brother saw his sister he felt desire for her. Unable to satisfy it, his teeth grew long and he became a demon. The sister was upset and tried to kill herself. Then the God Sakra intervened and took her up to his world, leaving the brother to become Kadavara, who from that day started to cause trouble for women. Especially when there is trouble with menstruation, it is caused by Kadavara dosa.

This story contains a number of elements which are common in the origin myths of Sinhalese demons (see Amarasingham 1978), particularly incest, uncontrolled desire, the vulnerability of women at menstruation, and violent revenge. Kadavara arises out of the vulnerability of a girl who is improperly shielded at her first menstruation and, as the story makes explicit, he is a man before he is a demon. In the broadest sense, the demon represents craving (*tanha*) and excess (*vädiya*) unchecked by social restraints.

The demon, then, is a multivalent symbol in Turner's (1967) sense. One pole is grounded in physiological processes, particularly those associated with fertility—such as sexual desire and the blood of menstruation and birth. The other pole represents mistakes—incest, marriage outside the group, violence toward children—which result from mistaken or excessive involvement in life processes. Demonic attack is a meaningful way for the Sinhalese to think about illness because it suggests that the body is not discontinuous with the social but interfused with it so that what goes wrong in a case like P.M.'s can be phrased in both social and physical terms simultaneously. The Kadavara diagnosis speaks to many aspects of P.M.'s situation—her femaleness, her infertility, her history of a negative experience at puberty. It links up with a whole constellation of cultural symbols surrounding these experiences—the associations between death, blood, and demons, the connection between Buddhist assumptions about suffering and the possibility of assuaging demonic affliction—to form part of what Good (1977) calls a semantic network, a web of meaning in which each term is related in some way to every other. Once established with this kind of potency, such a diagnosis is, I think, difficult to dislodge; certainly the biomedical treatment, which provided a paucity of symbolic connections, could not compete with it.

The Ritual Performance

G. performs two rituals derived from the *Kohomba Kankariya*, the *Väddi Yakun Pidīma* and the *Kadavara Pidīma*, as curing rituals for cases of demonically caused illness. Like other Sinhalese curing rituals, the *Kadavara Pidīma* provides an offering to the afflicting supernatural within a context of drumming, dancing, and dramatic performance. It is performed at night at the patient's house, before an audience of her relatives and friends. P.M.'s family was poor and the performance for her was therefore relatively simple, containing only the most essential elements. I will not go into detail about its content, which is nevertheless very complex, but will discuss those aspects of the ritual which are most relevant to her case, namely, its structure and its portrayal of the demonic.

Kapferer (1974) points out that most Sinhalese exorcism rituals have a two-part structure. The first section, which usually occurs before midnight, contains invocations, dances, and preparations which serve to emphasize the reality of the demonic world and the seriousness of its effect on human life. The second section, after midnight, consists of a number of dramatic episodes in which the demons are acted out in comic form and presented as increasingly ridiculous. Kapferer suggests that "overinvestment" in the idea of the demonic is one aspect of the patients' illness and that this is reduced through the medium of humor, which diminishes the psychological influence of the afflicting demons.

The *Kadavara Pidīma* which was performed for P.M. contained both serious and comic episodes. These did not occur in the order described by Kapferer, in that the humorous sections occurred quite early in the ritual.[6] The ritual had five major sections (I simplify this somewhat):

1. An altar (*aila*) was constructed along one wall of the patient's house with an offering table for Kadavara placed before it. The performance began about 8:00 P.M., with G. as chief *kattadiyā* presiding over a dancer, drummer, and assistant. The period before 10:30 consisted of invocations to the gods and demons, dances taken from the *Kohomba Kankāriya*, and a dance for the patient

based on a song in which Yasodhara laments the loss of Prince Siddhartha (the Buddha).

2. From 10:30 to midnight, joking dramas were performed. These are related to mythical themes of the *Kohomba Kankāriya* and do not contain a representation of Kadavara himself. In one a Väddi demon appears and others enact scenes from village life. The comic episodes make fun of the "wildness" of the demon, gradually "domesticating" him.

3. At midnight, an offering was made to Kadavara, consisting of various foods (including the "low" foods given only to demons and ghosts, such as burned meat). A live chicken was also offered. Kadavara was asked to take these foods and "remove all evils (*doṣas*)" from the patient.

4. At about 2:30 G. performed a *billa* or sacrifice. This is a "trick" on the demon in which the exorcist lies on a mat, chanting protective spells, and asks the demon to enter his body and leave the patient. It is thought that his magical power will protect him from harm, and that once the demon has been lured out of the body of the patient he will not be able to reenter because of the protective magic of the ritual. After G. had fallen into trance, the mat was rolled up and carried out of the house[7]; a few minutes later, he staggered back in, supported by his assistants. At the end of this episode, the patient gave a coin and betel leaf to G., and repeated "all evils will go away" (*siyalu dosa duruvenda*).

5. The early morning hours were taken up with protective rites and assurances that the affliction was over. An amulet was charmed and tied on the patient and a pot of milk was boiled (a symbol of fertility and good fortune). Once again the gods were invoked and thanked for their help. P.M. sat quietly, holding her baby, throughout the ritual. She did not go into trance, but watched carefully and laughed during the joking episodes. She told us that for her the most important part of the ritual was the moment when the demon entered the body of the *kaṭṭaḍiyā* (*billa*), at which point, she felt faint and broke out into a sweat. She is certain that Kadavara actually left her then.

The ritual then, has three parts : (1) affirmation of the demonic presence through invocation and dance, (2) negation of the power of the demon through humor and drama, and (3) affirmation of the demon through offerings and sacrifice intended to remove his influence. This structure mirrors the way in which the demon has been associated with the patient's life. In the patient's history the demon moves from being an uncontrolled presence, to being forestalled or held at bay by the vow, to being brought into controlled contact with the patient during the exorcism. In both history and ritual there is a pattern of increasing contact with and control over him. In the course of this contact Kadavara changes aspects several times, sometimes associated with the gods, sometimes frightening, sometimes stupid and 'blind' and sometimes an image of the inversion of social norms and meanings. This variation in his power is one of the transformative aspects of the combined action of the vow and ritual.

The fact that this ritual does not follow the sequence presented by Kapferer (1974) and, by placing the "funny" before the "scary" sections, deviates from the pattern described as standard by the *kaṭṭaḍiyā* himself, suggests not only a condensation in response to economic considerations, but also an adjustment of the ritual structure in response to the situation. That is, we can see a Sinhalese ritual as having numerous potential emphases depending on its use. Though the ritual is not changed to conform to an individual's specific circumstances, the totality of the ritual can address a number of different kinds of situations (this point is made by Obeyesekere 1977). In this performance confirmative rather than processual aspects are in focus. That is, the ritual unfolds, as Obeyesekere (1977) and Kapferer (1974) have made clear, in an explicit movement from involvement to detachment, toward the formation of a less intense relationship between the patient and the affliction. For the patient suffering from, say, prepsychotic symptoms, this processual aspect may be all-important. But the ritual also contains a number of episodes which emphasize that the affliction is *over*. Among these are the offering to the demon, the sacrifice (as suggested by the patient's statement that this was especially powerful in ending her relationship to Kadavara), and the final protective rites. All of these act on the end of the relationship with the demon, not through the subtle transformations of the joking episodes, but in terms of clear-cut images of removal and restraint. We can think of this kind of ritual as being like a prism, with the play of light varying depending on the angle held to view. The angle in this case emerges from the sense in which the diagnosis is being played out and laid to rest, rather than from the more transformative aspects of the ritual.

Discussion

Turning first to the question raised earlier—what makes this diagnosis "stick" in spite of the presence of other, competing diagnoses?—we can see that several aspects of the ritual sequence contribute to the permanence of the diagnosis.

1. The vow gives a provisional reality to the diagnosis, allowing healer and patient to "try out" an explanatory model featuring a particular demon by ritually linking demon and patient. While the vow is in effect it ties the patient and family to a particular way of looking at the illness and gives concrete form to generalized apprehension. It also sets up a relationship in time to the cause of the illness, by placing a time limit on the demon's incursions into the patient's life, and thus creating a frame within which the illness takes on meaning in relation to a specific cause. Because the vow "works," it gives concrete form and "sticking power" to the diagnosis.

2. There is a high correspondence in this case between the nature of the cause (diagnosis) and the nature of the illness. The Kadavara diagnosis, as we have shown, is symbolically powerful in its connection of demonic intrusion and reproductive problem. While P.M. made other vows in the course of her illness, these were to gods (reflecting, perhaps, a desire to start at the "top" in searching for cure) and did not have a comparable richness of connective links to the nature of the affliction.

When madness (*pissu*) is attributed to demonic possession, the possessed person confirms the diagnosis through her behavior, by entering trance and by responding appropriately to the actions of the healer. As Obeyesekere (1977) has shown, such cases can sometimes turn into a battle of wits between exorcist and patient as the patient struggles to maintain the advantages conferred by her diagnosis. In P.M.'s case, maintenance of this diagnosis is dependent on physical changes and the patient's role in shifting the focus onto the symbolic vehicle of the demon is more passive than in the case of madness. Thus the patient's condition and the characteristics of the diagnosis fit together independently of any direct action other than the vow.

3. It may seem obvious that when there is a cure, the diagnosis connected with it wil take on permanence and "reality" (Waxler 1977). While this is clearly a factor in this case, it should be noted that the diagnosis implicit in the Western treatment remained secondary in spite of its effectiveness. This was also true in the case previously reported, where the Western diagnosis did not count heavily among those presented (Amarasingham 1980). This suggests that while cure contributes to the stability of a diagnostic decision, it alone is not sufficient: the diagnosis must have other kinds of correlation with the patient's situation.

These aspects of the diagnosis—ways in which it "sticks" to the patient—suggest one way in which time is important here, as the medium through which the diagnosis takes on increasingly greater meaning and permanence. Time is also important in another, more puzzling way. What is striking about this case is the disarticulation between the timing of the treatment and the course of the illness. The illness and cure proceed along one dimension—the natural course of pregnancy and birth—while the vow and ritual unfold in their own time, corresponding to events in the patient's life but not lining up with the problem as it would be conceived in Western terms. Thus, the ritual itself gives no indication of the prior existence of the vow, and contains the same playing out of an on-going relationship with the demon as it would for any other illness for which it is performed. The playing out in ritual happens after the involvement of the patient is, in our sense, over. But for the patient the relationship to the demon has become the problem; it is no longer phrased as barrenness which has worked itself out in natural time, but as a negative connection to Kadavara which must be resolved in ritual time, that is, in ritual which need make no reference to time because it stands outside it. The illness, then, is not over with the birth of the baby, but only with the deliverance of baby and mother from an involvement which is threatening both to them.

Thus the crucial relationship is not between the course of the illness and its treatment, but between the affliction and its symbolic image. We see in this case that the distinction between diagnosis and treatment is an artifical one. The diagnosis is the treatment (that is, it corresponds to the period of the existence of the problem), and the treatment is "diagnostic" in the sense that it takes some of its meaning from its confirmation of the truth of the diagnosis.

The symbolic links between the patient's situation and the ritual formulation of it are made in time, but not in a time which unfolds lineally.

This suggests that there may be several ways in which symbolic forms and illness are connected in time, and that by assuming lineal relationships among cause, diagnosis, treatment, and cure, we miss some of the complexity and subtlety of ritual treatment. The following typology suggests itself:

1. In those cases which make up the vast bulk of the literature on this topic, there is a linear relationship between illness and the symbolic forms in which it is diagnosed and treated. The personal content of the illness (e.g. symptoms, connection to social role) is linked to a symbolic vehicle through diagnosis; this then becomes the form manipulated and played out in ritual. The symbolic transformation effected by the ritual is assumed to be paralleled in some way within the patient and the social network, resulting in change and cure. For example, in Obeyesekere's psycho-cultural exegesis the patient identifies her problems with mythical and demonic figures embodying certain aspects of her life; during the ritual performance, which occurs after this identification is well established, she acts out this relationship and experiences a resolution of the situation which was troubling her. While the symbolic associations are extremely complex, the timing is straightforward, moving from an initial tentative identification to increasing negative involvement (illness), climaxing in the ritual resolution (Obeyesekere 1977).

2. In contrast to this classic situation, there are other kinds of ritual treatment in which the patient's experience of the illness and the symbolic content of treatment are not in contact with one another at all. The curative effect inheres only in the process of seeking cure itself, not in a direct relationship between what the curer does and what the patient perceives to be wrong. For example, McCreery (1979) describes a form of Taiwanese curing ritual in which there is almost no contact between the patient and the healer. Patients bring problems to healers based on a bare-bones notion of "what is wrong", and the healers perform a ritual out of sight and hearing of the patient, with little or no explanation of what it means. A similar disjunction occurs when Chinese patients seek help from Western psychiatrists for symptoms which they consider somatic but which are perceived by the healer as psychological. In this case, the process of treatment (e.g. talking therapy) has no meaning to the patient, who continues to use his own system of explanation (Kleinman, Eisenberg, and Good 1978). In these cases, the only temporal link is a brief agreement that "something" is wrong; the diagnosis, however, unfolds differently for the patient than for the healer.

3. A different kind of situation develops when, instead of a paucity of symbolic understanding, there is a wealth of competing understandings. A number of symbolic systems may be built up together into an overlapping network of treatments in which none is discarded and none is made central. This results in a number of fleeting and perhaps tenuous relationships between what is wrong and the symbolic systems making sense of it. The passage of time, in this case, does not result in increased adherence to one diagnosis, but rather in an in-

creasingly flexible interpretation of the illness. This situation is described by me in an earlier paper (Amarasingham 1980) and alluded to by Waxler (1977) and Kunstadter (1975). Like the case presented here it requires a suspension of our linear understanding of time since it involves persistent contradiction and complexity during the entire course of illness and treatment.

4. Finally, there are cases like that presented in this paper where diagnosis is the major symbolic treatment during the course of the illness, carrying the weight of making sense of the illness until it is, in Western terms, ''over.'' In this case, the ritual performance manifests the meanings built up in the process of diagnosis, but disconnects them in time from resolution of the illness itself.

It is relatively easy to describe the first kind of situation, where diagnosis and treatment have a straightforward relationship in time, not in the sense that the intricacy of ritual process is easy to understand, but because the time-line along which such cure develops corresponds to our sense of how cure works. The other three situations contrast with our usual sense of how time, diagnosis, and affliction are related. Yet such anomalous situations probably make up a fair proportion of cases in many societies, including our own. They suggest that a lack of fit may be important, not only because these less straightforward connections between illness and treatment are interesting in themselves, but also because they can tell us something about how people think of the meaning of affliction in relation to time and causality.

NOTES

1   Although *yakās* or demons are ''supernatural'' in some senses of the English word, they are closer to humans than is suggested by our notion of the supernatural.

2   The *kotahalu* involves the ritual seclusion of the girl during her first menstruation, followed by a ritual bath performed by a washerwoman and the removal of all polluted materials from the house.

3   G. has not been consulted before because the family had been going to a specialist who lived near them (and who was probably less expensive).

4   G. said that the vow is performed three days after the start of menstruation, before the woman has had a bath. However, the family suggested that they went to see G. only after they realized that P.M. was pregnant.

5   It is unclear why P.M. went to a hospital for this pregnancy and not the others; probably this was the first time she got as far as the third month without a miscarriage. The combining of ritual and medical treatment described here is extremely common in Sri Lanka (see Amarasingham 1980).

6   This suggests the frustration inherent in trying to understand Sinhalese ritual as an unfolding in lineal time, since the constructions of the anthropologist may be much more consistent than those of the ritualist, for whom form and content are more readily merged.

7   Ideally the mat would be carried to a cemetery; in this case, it was carried to a crossroads not far from the house.

REFERENCES

AMARASINGHAM, Lorna Rhodes
    1978 "The Misery of the Embodied: Representation of Women in Sinhalese Myth." *In*
        Judith Hoch-Smith and Anita Spring (eds.), *Women in Ritual and Symbolic Roles*. New
        York: Plenum.
    1980 "Movement among Healers in Sri Lanka: A Case Study of a Sinhalese Patient."
        Culture, Medicine, and Psychiatry 4: 71-92.
ENGELHARDT, H. Tristram
    1974 "The Disease of Masturbation: Values and the Concept of Disease." *Bulletin of the
        History of Medicine* 48: 234-248.
GOOD, Byron J.
    1977 "The Heart of What's the Matter: the Semantics of Illness in Iran." *Culture,
        Medicine, and Psychiatry* 1: 25-58.
KAPFERER, Bruce
    1974 "First Class to Maradana: the Sacred and the Secular in Sinhalese Exorcism."
        Paper presented to the Berg Wartenstein Symposium. Wenner-Gren Foundation for
        Anthropological Research, No. 64.
KLEINMAN, Arthur M., L. EISENBERG, and B. GOOD
    1978 "Culture, Illness, and Care." *Annals of Internal Medicine* 88: 251-258.
KUNSTADTER, P.
    1975 "Do Cultural Differences Make Any Difference? Choice Points in Medical Systems
        Available in Northwestern Thailand. *In* Arthur Kleinman et al. (eds.), *Medicine in
        Chinese Cultures*. Washington, D.C.: NIMH, DHEW #75-653. Pp. 351-383.
McCREERY, John
    1979 "Potential and Effective Meaning in Therapeutic Ritual Culture." *Culture, Medicine,
        and Psychiatry* 3: 53-72.
OBEYESEKERE, G.
    1976 "The Impact of Ayurvedic Ideas on the Culture and the Individual in Sri Lanka."
        In Charles Leslie (ed.), *Asian Medical Systems*. Berkeley: University of California
        Press. Pp. 201-226.
    1977 "Psychocultural Exegesis of a Case of Spirit Possession in Sri Lanka." *In* V.
        Crapanzano and V. Garrison (eds.), *Case Studies in Spirit Possession*. New York: John
        Wiley. Pp. 235-294.
SICHERMAN, Barbara
    1977 "The Uses of a Diagnosis: Doctors, Patients, and Neurasthenia." *Journal of the
        History of Medicine and Allied Sciences* 32: 33-54.
TURNER, Victor
    1967 *The Forest of Symbols*. Ithaca: Cornell University Press.
WAXLER, Nancy
    1977 "Is Mental Illness Cured in Traditional Societies? A Theoretical Analysis." *Culture,
        Medicine, and Psychiatry* 1: 233-253.
YALMAN, Nur
    1967 *Under the Bo Tree*. Berkeley: University of California Press.
ZOLA, Irving K.
    1973 "Pathways to the Doctor: From Person to Patient." *Social Science and Medicine* 7:
        677-689.

Medical Anthropology and the Ethnography of Spirit Possession

PETER J. CLAUS

California State University at Hayward, Hayward, U.S.A.

On Defining Problems

ETHNOGRAPHIC RESEARCH over the past several decades has become increasingly problem oriented. There is a tendency in this sort of research to formulate models of a cultural phenomenon before the phenomenon is investigated. Indeed, the very problem is identified before the research is carried out. Research and description consist more or less of identifying features of the phenomenon with features of the proposed model. Verbal terms and behaviors are selectively chosen out of a large universe of similar forms, and are then translated in terms of the model. Causal relationships postulated in the model are used to explain terms and interaction in the phenomenon. Ability to do this not only demonstrates the efficacy of the model, but provides a scientific explanation of the phenomenon in that it appears to reduce a welter of particular facts from a large number of cultures to a smaller number of variables, usually having a more objective, naturalistic base. In this process of translating a particular phenomenon to a more generalized model, problem oriented research often finds it unnecessary to investigate the broad cultural context of the phenomenon in question. Problem oriented research is generally highly focused. Moreover, the focus is preset to take in pragmatic features: problem oriented research is closely allied with applied anthropology. There has been a wide-spread neglect of ethnography as an exploratory science, capable of discovering new perspectives with which to understand the human condition.

When the phenomenon of spirit possession is encountered in India it is usually regarded in the broad spectrum of medical problems.[1] It hardly seems to matter whether or not it is so defined in Indian systems of thought. In this regard, it might not be a bad idea to remind ourselves that Westerners have not always looked at possession that way. When early missionaries encountered possession cults in southern India they described this as a *religious problem*. Early accounts translated the various terms for the spirits in question as devils and demons.[2] The villagers were given to "devil worship" and "devil dancing." They were possessed by the Devil. We needn't labor over the gross inaccuracy of this translation of the phenomenon other than to note that the missionaries did give credence to the native belief in possession by a spirit agent. Where they differed with the natives was in the nature of the spirit involved.

I doubt that any serious anthropological study gives credence to the native claim that they are possessed by spirits, although we do sometimes acknowledge that we can proceed with the study "as if there were spirits." On the other hand, we still feel strongly obliged to recognize that some "real" experience is represented in their belief and behavior. We make a stab at apprehending that experience on the basis of our own understanding of similar behavior and beliefs in the West. Hence, our interpretation of the phenomenon as a medical problem, or, more neutrally, as an altered state of consciousness. Perhaps we do not see it in terms of religious behavior because rational Christianity in the West today is more concerned with sin and ethical behavior in the world, and not with ecstatic religious experience. But, more likely, as scientists, it is our usual approach to abnormal behavior to explain it in terms of biological foundations. Placing spirit possession in the conceptual area of medical problems leads us in that direction from the very outset. This approach is supported by reference to certain selected instances of possession. These are primarily cases of undesirable possession. It is supported by the observation in these cases that possession often starts with expressions of anguish and ends with a "cure." That seems a lot like the hoped for progression of Western psychotherapy.[3] Furthermore, in some instances, native terminology and classification of spirits identify them with abnormal health conditions: specific diseases, madness, epidemics and the like. Some aspects of many diseases, to put it slightly differently, are associated with the influence or intrusion of a spirit. But these instances are hardly sufficient to regard all instances of spirit possession as native medical practices and transfer the phenomenon to a medical paradigm. What is worse, to do so merely leads us away from what is ethnographically relevant, which is, the documentation of the process by which individual experience comes to be interpreted through a system of collective symbols.

The Ideology of Tulu Spirit Possession

There are dozens of words in Tulu which are used in the context of what I have been calling spirit possession.[4] The most usual are *bhūta pattuṇḍu* ("the spirit caught ...") and *mayṭu battuṇḍu* ("... came into the body"). Both verbs (*pattunu* and *barpunu*) have a large range of uses, entailing subtle contextual nuances and making them difficult to translate with regard to a specific experience. The verb *barpunu* ("to come"), for example, may be used to say "I will come to your house," "Good will come from that," "I will get angry (anger comes to me)," "I understand Tulu (Tulu comes to me)," and so on. Several verbs describe the physical appearance of the possessed (e.g. *kumbarunu*, "shaking") and the internal experience (e.g. *ersunu*, "rising"; also *barpunu*, here, I believe, with the meaning "arising" or "becoming").

In a ceremonial context possession is more usually referred to as *darśana*, "appearance, relevation." The English phrase used by my informants was "so and so had a *darśana*," although a more literal translation would have been the more ambiguous "*darśana* happened to so and so" (*arugu darśana ātuṇḍu*). The intensity of the possession—which is, incidentally, a frequently discussed matter, while whether a medium is "really" possessed, or not, is rarely questioned—is expressed in terms of *eḍḍe battuṇḍu* or *eḍḍe pattuṇḍu*) "it came (or caught) well."

The spirit in question may be one of a number of different categories: *bhūta, daiva, kule, prēta, sirikulu, cikku,* and others. They include spirits of cultural heroes, animal spirits, ghosts, and anthropomorphic divinities of various sorts. Several publications are available which list over 300 or so spirits.[5] Many spirits and categories of spirits have only vague identities, but the character of some is elaborately described in long oral narratives (*pāḍdana*) which describe their birth, "adventures", and death. These are spirits which tend to have a large cult following. Many other spirits are incorporated into these cults under specific conditions. The cults spirits are said to be able to control other spirits and command them to leave the body of a possessed person. The ritual relationships amongst these spirits constitute a vast subject, much too complex to pursue in this paper. However, it should be noted that a great deal of discussion revolving around an unexpected possession concerns the identification of the spirit and which of the cult spirits has the authority to command it to stop bothering the possessed.

The affliction caused by a spirit is usually described as *upadra*, "trouble." This term may be applied to certain cases of unwarranted possession, but more frequently it is used to label violent diseases brought about by spiritual attack on humans, animals or crops. It is also used to describe unusual and annoying events, such as mushrooms growing inside a house, as well as slow, persistent wasting diseases. In many of these circumstances there is considerable ambiguity as to whether the spirit is an external agent of affliction or whether his internal presence is the cause of the trouble. Some afflictions are said to be caused by the spirit's "touch" or "scratch."

It remains to be said that by no means are all instances of spirit possession regarded negatively. In cult ceremonies possession by the appropriate spirit is regarded as normal, legitimate and desirable. In other circumstances it is often precisely because the spirit cannot easily possess a person that the person suffers discomfort. Resistance on the part of the person or members of his/her family, uncleanliness (ritual pollution) of the body, existence of the influence of another spirit or a curse are the primary reasons why a spirit might have difficulty possessing its human vehicle. Possession is regarded as a normal means for a being of the realm of *māya* to make its presence or, more specifically, its needs, known in the world of *jōga* (living humans). What causes problems is generally human interference in these matters.

In Search of a Framework

In the past we have focused our attention on the emotional experience of possession. We have identified the phenomenon as a medical problem and have narrowly researched it in terms of a cause-and-effect paradigm which presumes that it has some sort of somatic starting point. There is little in terms or concepts used by the people to suggest this to be the case. For them it is a religious phenomenon; it has a spiritual origin. We look at the act as a medical problem because we take biological features to be more basic than cultural or ideological ones.

Attention to the terms people use to describe unusual experiences leads us in a direction to view it as they do. For the ethnographer this is a worthy goal. But reference to terminology of this sort is not the end of the line. It is only the beginning. The terms themselves—to come, to seize, to occur, appearance, spirit, trouble—are vague and metaphorical.[6] The verbs involved are all-purpose words, used in numerous contexts in general conversation. At best, here, they indicate that the transformation of character which the person undergoes is the result of the action of an external agent.[7] While that is an important part of the whole notion, it does not tell us specifically who the agent is, why it happens, why this person, why at this time, how, and so on. All of these questions are important to those people around the possessed person. Some of the answers are revealed after lengthy discussion and ritual action. The answers to some of the questions, however, are so deeply imbedded in the structure of the Tulu ideology that they are hardly ever raised. Many of the answers are to be sought in social contexts and social processes. Others are to be discovered in the character of the spirit and even by asking the spirit itself. And still others are to be deciphered from ritual action and symbolic expression. Terminology is but a very small, albeit initially important, part of a very large inquiry.

My own research has led me to the investigation of the way possession conjoins the individual (sometimes representative of a larger group or category of which he is a part) with his/her society's moral order. The sentiments from which possession springs (along this line of thinking) are no doubt common to all societies and are handled in many societies in different ways.[8] They arise under a number of situations, largely culturally conditioned, in which the individual feels himself outside of the order of moral expectations in which he has been conditioned to see himself. The specific Tulu expression of this crisis is in terms of the encroachment of beings from the domain of *māya* (the strange, mysterious, supernatural) on the domain of *jōga* (the ordinary, manifest and ordered world humans live in). Social groups larger than the individual too, in times of crisis, question, or even as a course of periodic routine, reassert the primacy of an ideal order over the exigencies (however they may arise) of individual and daily life. The phenomenon of spirit possession—or rather a tradition of spirit possession—can provide a symbolic medium through which the individual (or group) re-adjusts himself to an appropriate order.

This line of research does not preclude the validity or worthiness of studying other aspects of possession, such as the state of the possessed consciousness
or body or the characterization of the possessed mental state in Western
psychological terms, but differs from these in several important ways. One is
that it focuses on the relationship between the individual and society in the context of a web of moral expectations and responsibilities. It does not view the
possessed individual as necessarily *pathological* (although a particular society
may view the person as pathological) nor as involved in a conscious manipulation of others. Nor does it hope to uncover the purely personal experience of
possession.

Secondly, since the way the individual is related to his society in terms of a
moral system is expressed symbolically, this line of investigation, deals exten-
sively with the interpretation of the symbolic systems contained in myth and
ritual. That is to say, while studies of possession which concentrate on, say, the
psychological aspects tend to seek causal links in terms of Western scientific
knowledge of psychotic states, my own research has consisted of an investigation of how these sentiments are interpreted by and expressed in the symbolic
systems of South Indian culture.

The symbolic systems I have concentrated on are of two sorts: classification systems and models. In brief, classification provides order even where no
inherent differences and similarities can be perceived. It creates an order the
people of a culture accept. It serves them, among other ways, to know what to
expect from all those people and things which surround them. In this sense it is
a moral order. It importantly serves as a reference grid as well. Disruption of
order, inter-participation of elements or aspects of different classes, signal a
fundamental crisis for a people because an agreed upon set of expectations no
longer holds true. Of course, not all members of a group conceive exactly the
same order and, in fact, there are clearly many areas of a community's thought
where there are a variety of orders more or less contradictory to one another.
Concepts of order are portrayed through a number of different means
(metaphors, pictures, symbols, etc.) and each have a number of potentially different interpretations. In these areas there can be disagreement, argumenta-
tion or passive coexistence with regard to expectations. However, there are
other areas of communal thought in which a confusion of categories and expectations signal a more basic threat to man's imposed order. These are areas
upon which human existence itself, as perceived by a culture, is dependent.
For many Tulu-speakers one of these areas is the distinction between *māya* and
jōga. Since this distinction separates much of the mysterious, unseen and intangible from that which is human and humanly regulated, inter-participation
of the two categories is a serious threat to human existence. The distinction of
māya and *jōga* is of a high order and each category consists of a number of
subsets. The area of disturbance in the *jōga* class is readily apparent, but the
category of *māya* agents is often not easily discerned outside of a carefully controlled ritual context. It usually takes a diviner to ascertain this information.
Once the class of agents is known, procedures are put into use to isolate and
control the disruption and put the classification system back into order.

This is where models come into play. Models help people to conceive things in workable forms. Entities in the intangible, mysterious realm of *māya* are conceived on the model of a human. They are dealt with in the model of human relationships. Ritual is based on a model of a social situation. Even aspects of the classification of *māya* beings are based on models of social structure. The most important aspect of a model is not its static quality of picturing the relationships between things, as classifications are, but in providing a process for dealing with them. In the case of possession—the confusion of the realm of *māya* and *jōga*—the process is generally one of putting things back into order and restoring the normal expectations a community has agreed upon.

My interest in myth and ritual bear upon this process. But I hasten to point out that myth and ritual form only a part of the larger background in which most cases of possession take place. Even in Tuluva culture which appears to have one of the most elaborate sets of possession cult traditions in India, most possession is handled in a welter of impromptu contexts more directly studied through case histories and the collection of oral commentaries and less directly through the influence of standard myths and rituals. I assume, however, that myth and ritual traditions both encourage and help to frame the individual instances of possession and I have tried to demonstrate this in a number of cases (Claus 1973; 1975; 1978; 1979a; 1979b).

There is no doubt as to the importance of myth and ritual in cults in which possession is a regular feature of the ceremony in other areas of Southern India as well. In some cases recitation of myth (legend, epic, story) dominates the ceremony and possession occurs only at certain intense moments, usually associated with the hero(ine)'s valorous death, or at the point in the story during which the hero, loosed from the restraints of a normal order, confronts those who would seek its destruction. In other cases, the entire night-long, and even week-long, ceremonies are dominated by ritual performances punctuated by numerous instances of possession. In these cases, often possession of different intensity (e.g. the *vilu pattu* tradition of Nagarcoil described by Blackburn 1980) mark stages in the progressive "depth" dimension of the ritual, or possession passes from one set of personnel to another, as in the case of the Tulu *bhūta kōla* (Claus 1973). In these cases, also, a greatly foreshortened ritual version of the myth is associated with the ritual (cf. also Beck 1982), but the expanded versions must also be present in the participants' memory.

Not only "professional" religious specialists, but also "oridinary" members of the audience are occasionally drawn into the possession ritual in various degrees. Usually this form of possession is characterized by a mild, inarticulate trance state, but sometimes it takes the form of a violent (though often no more clearly articulated) frenzy. I am not aware, however, of any studies which explore the reasons why members of the audience become possessed although many reports mention the occurrence. My guess would be that this merely attests to the strength and intensity of the performance and its consistent structure which is designed to lead the participants into a deep level enactment of the heroes life (Blackburn 1980). It may be that the world of the spirit is not in any case very distant from the lived-in world of the villager.

There are certain instances in which "non-professional" possession is regular and elaborate in its expression. The several with which I am most familiar are found in Tulunad. In an earlier paper (1973), I described a case of possession among the audience attending an annual village *bhūta* ceremony. As is often the case during such ceremonies, village legal matters were discussed in the presence of the village spirits during the stage when the spirit possesses the body of the cult priest (*pūjari*). In the course of the proceedings a woman from one of the litigant's family was possessed by a household spirit, and this spirit then proceeded to argue the household's case. The woman began her possession with a frenzied trance, but was soon encouraged to come into more focused possession by the possessed priest. Possession brought the legal matter to the level of the spiritual realm and conjoined not only the village, but also the household, each through their possessed representative, to a moral order above the level of day-to-day interests.

Another example may be cited from the northern part of Tulunad in which a large proportion of the village "audience" routinely partakes in a variety of possession and trance forms at the annual village rituals. The ritual can be regarded as a sort of renewal rite in which members of the village individually and as respresentatives of groups express through possession states their relationship to the spiritual order which ideally governs the village:

> The village headman (he is still referred to by a royal title in the context of the ritual) is seated in front of the village temple along with the deity, who takes form in the body of a priest-medium. Women from each of the village households surround the pair and the women themselves become possessed by their household ancestors and spirits, who are considered to be in the village deity's retinue in the co-existent realm of māya, and who desire to be present at their lord's appearance during his "visit" to the realm of the living. After the headman pays his tribute to the deity, the men of the village file past the lords of the two realms, offering their loyalty and a small symbolic tribute. They receive in return the blessings of the royal pair and the promise of continued prosperity and protection. Women then walk barefoot through a pit of burning coals which has been constructed in front of the temple. In past times, it is said, the men performed acts of self-immolation to demonstrate their loyalty to the king and his deity. This act, on one hand, symbolizes the extremeties to which the men would go in the service of their lords, and on the other hand, the mystical protection from pain and injury the king and his deity could extend to those who serve them (Claus 1978: 31).

The Siri cult ceremonies provide an instance in which non-professionals are drawn into possession rituals in large numbers. Most participants have little contact with one another in their ordinary lives and many participants each year are newcomers. All have a history of troublesome individual possession previous to their participation in the cult, a condition which was resolved by their promise to serve (*sēve*) the Siri spirits as possession vehicles in subsequent years. At the annual Siri cult ceremonies the participants, mostly women, gather in small groups (some of which meet occasionally at a village shrine under the leadership of a male priest at other times in the year) and recite a ritual version of the legend of Siri. Soon all are possessed in one form or another. The attention of the adepts is given to helping novices to more easily and fully express the character of their possessing spirit. The violent, troublesome nature of the novice's possession is felt to be due to her inability to allow the spirit to fully possess her, and this is in turn due to either ineptitude on her part, or malicious resistance, often using mystical means, on the part of her relatives. A variety of means are used to facilitate her full possession. The ritual location, chanting the Siri legend, possession enactment of key episodes of the legend, the presence of possessed adepts and their use of kinship idiom to invite the novice into a spirit group, the power of the male priest to remove mystical obstructions, and so forth, all serve powerfully to encourage the novice to express her possession more articulately and elaborately in an accepted character. In short, recitation of myth and ritual action are brought together in a dramatic model through which the individual is reintegrated into a moral order.

We have seen then how ritual encourages and shapes the possession experience. In standard, periodic cult ceremonies the structure of the ritual performance and the formal recitation of myth easily transform the specialist into a spirit and the ceremony into an enactment of the exploits of a culture hero. Others may be drawn into performance as well, and in certain instances may be regularly encouraged to fully express their possession by means of a variety of ritual aids.

What it is that they are drawn into is often most clearly seen in myth. This is especially true in cases where the possessed embodies one of the many ''historic'' culture heroes. This sort of possession tends to be both more elaborate and more intense. The imagination of the South Indian villager finds its most elaborate and creative expression in the lives of the one-living heroes. Often these are based on real historic personages. However, there can be little question that the bulk of legends and epics consists of stylized elaboration of imagery already a part of oral tradition and everyday speech. The number of epics and legends of this sort in the different regional cultures of southern India is vast and many of the individual pieces are enormous in length. Collection and assessment of this body of literature has barely begun.

Scholars from different disciplines have viewed these works of oral tradition from a number of perspectives. However, most pertinent for the study of the relationship between these heroic epics and legends and their enactment in the form of possession is the ''moral imagination'' these works exhibit. In this it is not unlike the oral tradition of many cultures. Beidelman, for example, writes of Kaguru (an East African Society):

> Instead of considering situations and persons inextricably linked to a totality of phenomena over a long, even enduring, period of time, as in real life, the Kaguru story teller presents an extreme and limited case ... While stories avoid the complexities of possibilities in these daily problems, they do point out implications and difficulties posed as one tries to succeed where conflicting and competing loyalties perplex people, and where yesterday's enemies may be tomorrow's friends. Their very simplicity gives stories their attraction, just as the simplicity of sociological models both reduces yet helps explain a social reality. ... These stories are odd, not in the sense that they do not represent recognized characteristics, feelings, motives and roles, but in the sense that, whereas in real life these cannot all be proper-

ly judged and met by the same person or in one situation, here they are clearly defined and resolved (Beidelman 1980: 33).

Like Kaguru tales, the morality of South Indian oral traditions is not easy to discern, because the rightness or wrongness of the heroes' actions is conditioned by the circumstances. The Tulu legends, for example, relate the heroes' actions in desperate situations and what in the legends are regarded as courageous acts are often actions which would be at odds with the expectations of everyday life. Nor is the moral order abstractly, or directly, described. Instead it forms a set of assumptions, a backdrop against which the actions of the hero are tried in a series of dialectic relationships, and through which he emerges a hero.

There is a lot in common between the legends and the immediate lives of the possessed. Specific similarities can be found at all levels: structure, theme, mood, character, setting, action, etc. The legendary heroes provide a model for the possessed. Through the lives of heroes, in the limited and extreme contexts of their legends, people can find possible definition and resolution of their own circumstances. The fact that the heroes are medial beings—apotheosized humans—who define their heroism in desperate situations homologous to the situations living people are apt to be disturbed by, facilitates identification and transposition of their character. This is so not only in regular cult ceremonies, but also for those who experience desperate situations in their daily lives. Material I collected on reasons why many Tulu women are attracted to the Siri cult, where their initially vague, disturbing possession is brought toward resolution, suggested the following observations:

> The individual struggles to live with a condition which is threatening to her propitious conduct, upon which, in turn, the prosperity and reputation of those around her depend. The threat is almost invariably brought about by the lack of male protection which the cultural ideology requires in order that women may be secure against the ravaging intrusion of supernatural and human enemies. ... Under such precarious conditions a woman is vulnerable not only in the material world in which she must have sustenance, but also in the supernatural realm in which she is defenseless. By giving herself as a vehicle for one who might be her savior, a spirit of one who had preserved the concept of feminine virtue in her own lifetime, a woman chooses the lesser of two dangers. By becoming the vehicle of her spiritual protectress, she brings resolution to vague fears and apprehensions. The more clearly her tutelary spirit can be defined as virtuous, the more secure and powerful can be the woman's defense against those who seek to destroy her (Claus 1979: 49).

Conclusion

My argument in this paper is that the incidence of spirit possession is a complex ethnographic phenomena. To interpret it with a simplistic Western, medical paradigm is insufficient. There is no doubt that the possessed individual exhibits interesting abnormal psychological behavior and, further, that his or her actions often symbolically express in some way unresolved past experiences of an interpersonal nature. But this is largely expressed and interpreted in a culturally specific symbolic system and the individual is reintegrated into a moral community through ritual action. When we approach the phenomena through problem-oriented paradigms we short-circuit the ethnographic process. If we are to carry the investigation further we have to be careful that we touch base at all times with native concepts. Indigenous terms and metaphors point us in the right direction. Indigenous classification constitutes the landscape. Myth and ritual provide us with models of how people think about and experience what we are unable to observe.

This procedure will, I believe, lead us in a different direction than does the problem oriented research of medical anthropology. Problem oriented research of the sort I characterized in the beginning of the paper has a tendency to lead us back to where we started. We learn nothing new, nothing from others and little of real usefulness about ourselves. According to these views spirit possession is universally associated with specific psychological or physical conditions (e.g., calcium deficiency in the diet, as one recent suggestion runs). The behavior of the possessed is equated with the behavior of patients with such conditions. Ritual treatment of the possessed, to the extent that it is effective, is seen as a primitive form of the treatment of patients in a modern scientific clinic. These views ignore most of what is ethnographically relevant. We feel secure, perhaps, in identifying a universal or biological basis for behavior and confident in our own progressiveness for treating scientifically what others do with magic and ritual. But what do we really learn?

Unfortunately, possession is often ignored even in the ethnographies of cultures in which it occurs with remarkably high frequency and even in ceremonies in which the ethnographer records its occurrence. At best we are given a simple description of the possession behavior, or the costume, or the dancelike movements of the possessed, or the occurrence of the act in relation to the temporal and musical aspects of the ceremony. Almost nowhere do we find an investigation of the meaning of possession in the same sense as we find discussions of other major religious phenomena, such as sacrifice or witchcraft.

So far, ethnography has failed to bring to bear on this phenomena what is important from a larger cultural perspective. Ethnographers have missed an opportunity to understand a rather remarkable set of cultural events, a set which only the ubiquitous ethnographer is apt to witness in its greatest variety of forms and contexts.

What is probably most significant about possession is that it allows us to witness in detail the relationship between the expressive, and the interpretative and the integrative aspects of religion. Each case of possession is a case in point, varying from the highly standardized, routine and collective rituals held periodically at the village level to the spontaneous occurrence of possession in the household in the midst of daily life. The whole range is linked through a tradition of possession belief from which individual instances are interpreted and to which they contribute. We know little about such religious processes in any religious context, and a study of possession from this perspective would seem to me to constitute a major contribution.

NOTES

1   A classic example of this may be seen in Carstairs and Kapur 1976. There possession is
     treated as a psychiatric symptom along with other such symptoms as anxiety, depression,
     psychosis, etc. True, they do place it in the context of the local South Kanara cultural set-
     ting (e.g., pp. 59-61, 67-69) and qualify it as other than a mere symptom of mental illness
     by allowing that there is "... a close association between cultural beliefs and
     psychopathology ..." in the case of possession (1976: 110).
     A far more sophisticated discussion of the relationship between private symbols and public
     symbols having both personal and interpersonal significance may be found in
     Obeyesekere's recent book, *Medusa's Hair* (1981). In this book—too tightly argued and in-
     tricately documented to review here—Obeyesekere successfully demonstrates that
     phenomena such as possession can have deeply motivated unconscious meaning for the in-
     dividual and at the same time fit meaningfully into a network of religious ideology. The two
     approaches (the public and the private) and the two interpretations (psychological and
     religious) need not be viewed contradictorily, as I, also, argue later in this paper.
2   Defining the spirits worshipped by the Tuluvas as demons did not prohibit the 19th century
     missionary from studying the religious literature or practices of "demon worshipers," but it
     did, certainly, influence the way they treated the data. The Rev. A. Manner, for example,
     wrote in the preface to his fine collection of *pāḍḍana* (1886):
     "As the physician in the course of his study requires in many cases to apply himself to
     unpleasant research, even so does the Mission-worker require often to study adverse
     literature, which may not be pleasant, to enable him efficiently to cope with the difficult task
     of meeting the heathen on his own ground. From a scientific point of view these stories are
     not of much worth, but they serve to give one an insight into the hollowness of demon-
     worship and enable the Mission-worker among this class of people to gain an insight into
     their ideas and to follow out their line of thought. ... It is therefore in the interest of the
     Mission-worker to whom, as aforesaid, such information is peculiarly valuable, and not
     with any intent to give wider publication to these stories that we have had them printed and
     I have in hand a small number of copies for sale at cost-price to missionaries and Mission-
     workers only, strictly prohibiting the loan or sale of such under any circumstances what-
     soever, to the heathen" (1886: i).
3   There are, of course, other aspects of the relation between this class of spirits and the human
     realm which could lead us to assume that spirit possession is essentially a medical
     phenomenon. In popular belief all around South Asia, diseases of many types are associated
     with the supernatural (smallpox with Māri or Sitala; leprosy with the cobra, etc.). Propitia-
     tion of supernatural agents of disease is a common means of ridding the community or the
     individual of many types of disease. There is no doubt here that many South Asians adhere
     to a medical belief system which falls into the broad class of what George Foster calls a per-
     sonalistic etiology (Foster 1976; Foster and Anderson 1978). What is dangerous in this sort
     of labeling exercise, is to assume that the "real" diseases we recognize and explain by scien-
     tific medicine correspond to the same diseases another culture recognizes and explains by
     supernatural agents. If this were true, medical anthropology would have a rather simple
     task of translating one system into another. But this is not often the case. Not only are there
     different (from ours) and subtly varied notions of causality involved in any one system, but
     there are different ranges of phenomena identified as diseases. The very ideas of what con-
     stitutes disease, health, etc., are different. There are, for example, what Obeyesekere calls
     "cultural diseases," because "they are created, at least partly, by the cultural definition of
     the situation" (Obeyesekere 1976: 207).
4   For more details, see Nichter's (1979) extensive discussion of the vocabulary of illness in
     this region of India.
5   See Padmanabha 1971; Bhatt 1975; Burnell 1894.
6   I am referring here to metaphor in the sense discussed in the book *Metaphors We Live By*, by
     Lakoff and Johnson (1980).
7   The most usual general concept of the body which the metaphors for possession entail is that

of a container. In this respect, the body is likened to an idol or a temple, both of which are also containers for the supernatural. Pots, stones, trees, poles, and seats (benches, swings) are also common "containers" for spirits and deities. Each of these items, including the body, emphasizes somewhat different aspects of the notion of containing: temples, for example, often stress a series of boundaries; idols stress visual form; long, flexible poles allow the vitality of the spirit contained therein to be expressed through a violent undulating motion. The human body, having a number of these features, is thought to be an especially appropriate container for the spirits of cultural heroes and deceased kinsmen.

8 For a listing of comparative material on spirit possession in other cultures, see Bourguignon 1968a, 1968b, 1973, 1976. Bourguignon uses mental and physical states as the basis for ordering her data.

REFERENCES CITED

BECK, B. E. F.
  1982 *The Three Twins: The Telling of a South Indian Folk Epic.* Bloomington: Indiana University Press.
BEIDELMAN, T. O.
  1980 "The Moral Imagination of the Kaguru: Some Thoughts on Tricksters, Translation, and Comparative Analysis." *American Ethnologist* 7: 27-42.
BHATT, P. G.
  1975 *Studies in Tuluva History and Culture.* Manipal (India): Manipal Power Press.
BLACKBURN, S.
  1980 "Performance as Paradigm: A Rhythm in a Tamil Oral Tradition." Paper presented at the conference on Models and Metaphors in Indian Folklore, Berkeley, California, February 7-10, 1980.
BOURGUIGNON, E.
  1968a "World Distribution and Patterns of Possession States." *In* R. Prince (ed.), *Trance and Possession States.* Montreal: R. M. Bucke Memorial Society.
  1968b "A Cross-Cultural Study of Dissociational States: Final Report." Columbus: Ohio State University Research Foundation.
  1973 "Introduction: A Framework for the Comparative study of Altered States of Consciousness." *In* E. Bourguignon (ed.), *Religion, Altered States of Consciousness, and Social Change.* Columbus: Ohio State University Press.
  1976 *Possession.* Corte Madera, California: Chandler and Sharp.
BURNELL, A. E.
  1894 "The Devil Worship of the Tuluves." *Indian Antiquity* 23.
CARSTAIRS, G. M. and R. L. KAPUR.
  1976 *The Great Universe of Kota.* London: The Hogarth Press.
CLAUS, P.
  1973 "Possession, Protection, and Punishment as Attributes of the Deities in a South Indian Village." *Man in India* 53:231-242.
  1975 "The Siri Myth and Ritual: A Mass Possession Cult of South India." *Ethnology* 14: 47-58.
  1978 "Heroes and Heroines in the Conceptual Framework of Tulu Culture." *Journal of Indian Folkloristics* 1: 28-42.
  1979a "Spirit Possession and Spirit Mediumship from the Perspective of Tulu Oral Traditions." *Culture, Medicine, and Psychiatry* 3: 29-52.
  1979b "Mayndala: A Myth and Possession Cult of Tulunad." *Journal of Asian Folklore Studies*: 38-95-129.
FOSTER, G.
  1976 "Disease Etiologies in Nonwestern Medical Systems." *American Anthropologist* 78: 773-782.
FOSTER, G. and B. ANDERSON
  1978 *Medical Anthropology.* New York: John Wiley and Sons.

LAKOFF, G. and M. JOHNSON
    1980   *Methaphors We Live By*. Chicago: University of Chicago Press.
MANNER, A.
    1886   *Pāḍḍanolu*. Mangalore: The Basel Mission Press.
NICHTER, M.
    1979   "The Language of Illness in South Kanara (India)." *Anthropos* 74: 181-201.
OBEYESEKERE, G.
    1976   "The Impact of Ayurvedic Ideas on the Culture and the Individual in Sri Lanka."
           In Charles Leslie (ed.), *Asian Medical Systems*. Berkeley: University of California
           Press. Pp. 201-226.
    1981   *Medusa's Hair*. Chicago: University of Chicago Press.
PADMANABHA, P.
    1971   "Special Study Report on Bhuta Cult in South Kanara Distrtict." Census of India,
           Series 14 Mysore (Karanataka), Miscellaneous (a). Delhi: Government of India
           Press.
ROGHAIR, G.
    1978   "The Role of Brahma Nāyudu in the Epic of Palnadu." *Journal of Indian Folkloristics*
           1: 15-26.

Desire in Bengali Ethnopsychology

DEBORAH P. BHATTACHARYYA*

De Pauw University, Greencastle, U.S.A.

T HIS PAPER IS PART OF EXTENDED RESEARCH conducted in Bengal in 1975-76 on folk conceptions of mental illness. Here I shall explore the Bengali belief that excessive desire can have destructive consequences for the individual. Conceptions of *paglami* (madness) highlight the harmful role of frustration, when desires cannot be gratified. Furthermore, this belief is echoed in the classical Sanskrit literature and throughout other areas of Bengali culture. It can also be seen in the work of G. S. Bose, the Bengali founder of a variant of psychoanalysis. From this data, I shall identify two themes and then demonstrate how they can be integrated into a common framework wherein *paglami* serves as a category of deviance which illustrates Bengali conceptions of the nature of human beings and the relationship between human beings and the surrounding environment.

One of the basic questions of my research has been "What is *paglami*?" Before I present one of the answers to this question, I want to identify the theoretical orientation which I have used in formulating such an answer. In order to determine what *paglami* is, it is necessary to delineate the moral meanings constructed by actors in the situated context of their behavior. When Bengali actors identify a particular phenomenon (behavior, event, individual, etc.) as being *paglami*, they are communicating to others that certain moral meanings and a certain theory of the world apply to that phenomenon. They are saying that the phenomenon possesses the property of "*paglami-ness*" and therefore it becomes constituted as a particular kind of social object. The properties which are conferred upon the phenomenon by virtue of this labeling process comprise the concept and theory of *paglami*. Thus, in order to discover what *paglami* is, it is necessary to formulate that theory and to establish the properties which are asserted through the application of the label *paglami*.

Probably the most important characterization of *paglami* is that it is deviance. Deviance refers to a property conferred upon behavior by a social audience in order to indicate that it is outside the cultural boundaries of the group (Erikson 1966: 6ff.). As such, it is a property of behavior which stimulates a reaction serving to indicate that the behavior is judged as inappropriate, immoral, or otherwise not in accordance with the normative expectations which

* *Acknowledgments.* This paper is based on research supported by grants from the Social Science Research Council and the American Institute of Indian Studies, 1975-1977.

apply in that particular context. Thus, to formulate the theory of *paglami* we have to examine the ways in which *paglami* is deviance, the ways in which *paglami* deviates from the normative expectations which Bengalis have of each other. If "social groups create deviance by making the rules whose infraction constitute deviance" (Becker 1963: 9), then *paglami* is best defined by locating those rules which generate *paglami*, those boundaries which it transgresses. As Erikson (1966) has noted, interaction surrounding deviance communicates to the members of a community where the boundaries lie and thus establishes the cultural space within which the group is located. Thus, to delimit a particular deviant category such as *paglami* is a means by which that cultural space can be identified. By examining *paglami* as deviance, we can establish the cultural relevance of the psychiatric domain as a border area which informs of the cultural territory that lies within. In this paper, I hope to show that *paglami* as a deviant category depends upon particular theories of the nature of human beings and especially the relationship between human beings and the surrounding environment.

The Destructive Consequences of Frustrated Desire

In an earlier paper (Bhattacharyya 1977), I noted that the major etiological factor involved in *mathar golmal* (head malfunctioning) is "shock." Here I want to examine this concept more closely. In addition to case histories obtained from relatives of mental patients, I asked over ninety lay Bengalis to tell me why people become *pagol* (see Table I). The English word "shock" and the Bengali term *aghat* are both frequently used. *Aghat* is perhaps best translated as "a heavy blow" and can be used to refer to either mental or physical blows. Other commonly used terms are *śok* (grief, mourning), *dukkho* (sorrow), *cinta* (worry), *ɔbhab* (insufficiency), and *manośik dondo* (mental conflict).

All of these terms as well as the examples used by informants, indicate that certain emotional states are likely to produce *paglami*. Specifically, these emotional states all seem to point to frustration as a key cause. This frustration may be economic (money worries), academic (failure in exams), career (lack of advancement), or emotional (unrequited love). Thus, as several respondents have noted, being unable to obtain what is deeply desired is the source of frustration. The most extreme example of such frustration and the one most frequently cited is *śok* (intense grief) where the death of a loved one prevents the fulfillment of one's desires. Thus, the primary attribute of "shock" is an emotional response to an extremely frustrating situation. The gratification of desire is prevented by some obstacle against which one's own efforts are totally ineffectual. In such a situation, the individual's wants, needs, and desires find no outlet, and to quote one respondent, they cross the limits of endurance. The image which comes to mind is the almost physical accumulation of emotion and thus the generation of intense pressure.

Table 1

Some Sample Responses to the Question: Why Does One Become Pagol?

1. *From mourning (śok)*, from insufficiency (ɔbhab) or getting a lot if one studies a lot, one becomes *pagol* (LC 6).*
2. When depression (*mon kharap*) happens, one becomes *pagol*. When someone does whatever he wants, one becomes *pagol* (LC 17).
3. If one worries, because of money or illness, one becomes *pagol*. If a shock (*aghat*) strikes the head hard, then one will become *pagol* (LC 23).
4. For many reasons. Because of poverty. If one fails when studies are good, one will become *pagol*. If "shock" is received, one will become *pagol*. If a lot of medicine is taken, one will become *pagol*. If the head becomes hot from sorrow (*dukkho*), it happens ... Many become *pagol* from "love affairs" (MC 4).
5. If one worries a lot about some little thing ..., if one thinks intensely about it, *mathar golmal* can happen. If there is some "deficiency", *mathar golmal* happens. "If he wants something but can't get it" (MC 6).
6. If one receives a lot of sadness (*dukkho*), one will become *pagol*. When the sadness crosses the limits of endurance, then one will become *pagol* (LC 29).
7. It happens from "shock"; if the only child dies. If, from shock (*aghat*), the body's "vital force" becomes less; if an "accident" happens; if there is "pressure" on the "brain" (MC 15).
8. If one receives a "shock"; if someone dies; if one suddenly receives a lot of money; because of family troubles (*jala*) (MC 16).
9. Hereditary. If one is sick. If one doesn't get something wanted wholeheartedly, one becomes *pagol* — be it consciously desired or unconsciously. One becomes *pagol* after taking medicine (MC 18).
10. One cannot adjust with one's own mind. If this conflict becomes "extreme", one's head becomes bad. If one worries a lot - from insufficiency, fear, domination (MC 19).
11. Someone wants something, "wants it desperately", but didn't get it (MC 21).
12. Perhaps in his mind, he wanted something, but didn't get it. If a man wants something a lot but doesn't get it, he becomes unhappy (ɔsanti), the mind breaks (*mon bheŋe pɔre*) and he becomes *pagol* (D 3).

* Letters and numbers in parentheses refer to the codes assigned to each respondent. Responses are translated from the Bengali; words or phrases in quotes were spoken in English.

This analysis is reinforced by the common belief that *paglami* can be cured if the desires of the individual are met. Marriage is almost universally recommended for an unmarried patient. The patient's need for both affection and sex will thereby be satisfied. In a Bengali newspaper article (*Ananda Bazar Patrika*, August 4, 1975), the reporter comments about one patient that "she might fully recover if she can get her boy friend back." Also, having a baby is thought to cure mental illness. One infertile patient told me that she was sure that all her problems would disappear as soon as she got pregnant. Basically, it is important to remove one's worries and the source of one's frustration so as to regain mental health. Perhaps this view is also responsible for the tremendous gentleness with which patients were often treated by family members.

The concept of "shock" points to the belief that excessive desire can have destructive consequences for the individual. The emphasis is on the harmful role of frustration, when desires cannot be gratified. This theme is echoed throughout other areas of Bengali culture. I want to begin by noting the view of desire found in the classical Sanskrit literature and then examine some additional ethnographic material. Finally, I shall comment on the work of G. S. Bose, the Bengali founder of a variant of psychoanalysis.

Even as early as the Upanishads, the idea is introduced that passion inhibits self-realization and that salvation (liberation, *moksha*) is dependent on a state of non-attachment. Thus, self-realization can occur only "when all the desires that dwell within the human heart are cast away ... when all the knots that fetter the heart are cut asunder" (from the Katha Upanishad, quoted in Murphy and Murphy (1968: 59). The liberated man has abandoned his worldly attachments and is free from desire or passion. Passion, as the motivational force which connects the individual to the objects of the environment, causes man's attachment to the phenomenal world, thereby impeding spiritual release.

In the Bhagavad Gita, passion is linked with *rajas* (energy, activity), one of the three *gunas* or attributes. Much of the Gita contrasts *sattva* action or the performance of *dharma* (duty) with *rajas* action or the expression of *kama* (passion). As de Bary notes (1958: 276), "Action, as such, is not detrimental to one's attainment of his spiritual goal. It is only one's attachment to the fruits of action" that prevents liberation. Salvation is still associated with the control of passion and of the senses so as to sever the Self's attachment to the world. The description of the self-realized individual is a portrayal of one whose desires have been extinguished (Bhagavad Gita, 2.55-71, quoted in Rao 1962: 179-80):

> He is known as one with equipoise (*sthitaprajna*, equanamity) when he eschews all overmuch desire and learns to be satisfied with himself. Difficulties disturb him not and pleasures fail to tempt him; freed from longing, dread and hate he is a sage with steady mind. His heart is settled in nothing, meeting good or evil he is neither happy nor sad. His senses are withdrawn, like the limbs of a turtle and his mind is steady. Objects of lust, unfed, disappear. ... Senses indeed are naughty and snatch the mind away. The wise one controls them all ... for when they are controlled, mind can be steady. Brooding over objects of enjoyment, one gets fixed on them; being fixed he craves for them. Craving (unfulfilled) leads to anger, and anger to confusion; confusion makes for unreasonableness and that results in madness, which is the road to destruction. Bereft of love and hate, senses bridled by the self, the individual obtains calmness. In calmness so all cares and worries find their end; calmness helps the mind settle. ... When mind yields to the whims of senses, it is led hopelessly astray, like a boat on water wafted by the gale.

From this perspective, it is especially interesting that attempts have been made to establish the relevance of yoga for the treatment of mental disturbances (Coster 1934; Deshmukh 1972; Goyeche 1972; Joshi 1964; Vahia 1969; Vahia *et al*, 1966, 1972, 1973a, and 1973b; Brar 1970; Masson 1974; Pal 1971; Jacobs 1961). Vahia, for instance, has attempted to formulate an explicit therapy based on yogic principles. He begins by noting that an individual's equilibrium can be disrupted by "disturbing thoughts ... associated with Raga (emotional attachment to appealing objects) or Dvesha (hatred or jealously towards ... objects ...)'' (Vahia 1969: 7). The goal of therapy is to help the patient become less affected by such disturbing thoughts. "He would now appreciate that his preoccupation with the maintenance of self-esteem was primarily responsible for his inadequate adjustment" (Vahia 1969: 10). By decreasing the importance of his egoistic self-esteem, the patient will be able to eliminate the disturbing thoughts, to concentrate on objective goals, and to become independent of environmental responses to his behavior which would otherwise cause stress and anxiety.

This belief in the destructive potential of passion is also evident in the common somatic complaint of extreme weakness and lethargy attributed to the loss of semen (see Carstairs 1956; Obeyesekere 1976). Semen is one of the seven *dhatu* (body substances) of Ayurvedic theory and it is generally believed that a man has a fixed amount of semen. Not only is this reserve reduced during ejaculation, but semen can "curdle" and "leak." Since semen is seen as the main source of a man's energy and power, any contamination or loss of semen is identified with a loss of strength. Carstairs (1956), on the basis of Rajasthani data, suggests that the cultural ideal, complete restraint from sexual activity, is generally compromised by subordinating sexuality to the service of *dharma* (duty)—satisfying one's wife and begetting children. Furthermore, he notes that the conservation of semen is associated with one's ability to achieve liberation. Since semen provides the energizing force of the individual, its preservation and channelization facilitates self-realization and final liberation. This conceptualization is a more concretized version of the Sanskritic belief that salvation requires the control of passion.

Turning to other ethnographic material, I want to examine certain child-rearing practices in Bengal. Western observers often comment on the "spoiling" of the Indian child. And indeed, it often appears that the major responsibility of other family members is to gratify the child's every whim (see Carstairs 1957; Spratt 1966; Kakar 1978). A baby is seldom allowed to cry for long, at least not without repeated efforts to soothe him/her. "Demand" nursing is the normal pattern and weaning is not only slow and gradual but often delayed until well into the second or even third year. Toilet training is accomplished with a minimum of harshness. As Surya (1968: 388) has commented, "A child rarely is exposed to the need to wait for anything or to stand any frustration for long. Any educative frustration of a child attempted by one member of the family is soon mollified by the over-protective attention of another." The most basic child-rearing rule seems to be: Minimize frustration by gratifying all desires.

The two major exceptions to this generalization—situations involving feeding and school studies—simply go to reinforce this conclusion. From an early age, all three of the bottle-fed babies with whom I was familiar were forced to drink all their milk. If the bottle was not finished, the milk was fed forcibly with a spoon, in spite of protesting cries. At later ages, toddlers would still be forced to eat. However, such coercion was definitely a last resort; mothers and other family members might spend a full hour cajoling the child to eat with distractions, bribes, and threats. And when force was finally adopted, it was with a great deal of anxiety. Thus, while coercion was used, there was a tacit recognition that it was only acceptable given the essential nature of eating. The second exception was the conflict over school studies. It was assumed that school children had to be made to study, and again, family members spent considerable time helping them with homework or just nagging them to get their studies done. Again, the use of force was not free of anxiety but was justified by the desire to see their children do well in school. These exceptions single out parents' basic obligations to the child—to help the child grow healthy and to enable him or her to learn.

One of the rationales behind such gratification of the child is the need to encourage the child's even-temperament (*thanda mejaj*). Deprivation causes frustration and anger and this predisposes the child to a greater likelihood to become frustrated and angry again. A vicious circle sets in. On the one hand, the child is believed to have little tolerance for frustration; on the other, early deprivation can have a lasting effect on the personality by making the child "hot-tempered" (*gɔrum mejaji*). Thus, "spoiling" the child precludes any frustration and thus preserves the child's emotional stability.

Another example of the belief in the necessity to satisfy desires is the *śad* ritual. This ritual is performed after the seventh month of pregnancy and before the birth of the child. The primary aim of the occasion is to ensure that the pregnant woman has all her wishes fulfilled. Indeed, *śad* means "desire" and is used in colloquial Bengali to indicate an intense longing or craving. In modern Bengal, the *śad* ceremony involves a feast at which guests present the woman with saris and sweets, both luxuries for all but the well-to-do. Interestingly, one Westernized Bengali woman who had dispensed with the traditional *śad* told me that her *śad* consisted of a dinner at a Chinese restaurant because she had been craving Chinese food. Indeed, specific food cravings are expected during pregnancy and, independent of the *śad*, attempts are usually made to provide the desired foods. The rationale behind this practice is that unfulfilled desires could be injurious to both mother and child: *śad* ensures an easy delivery and a healthy, happy (*thanda mejaji*) baby.

In addition to *mathar golmal* (head malfunctioning), possession and sorcery are also linked to mental illness and they too involve frustrated desire. A *bhut* (ghost) is a disembodied self which has not obtained release so that it can proceed to the next life. Persons who die through *ɔpoghat mritu* (unnatural death), that is, those who die "before their time," are particularly likely to become *bhut*. *Bhut*, then, are the selves of persons whose death does not entail their detachment from the world of the living, which is especially the case of persons whose death comes before they are able to live out their life in full. This residual attachment to the world of the living is apt to occur if the individual dies without having satisfied important passions. An unmarried man (and therefore one who is presumed not to have satisfied his sexual passions) and a childless woman are prime candidates for becoming *bhut*. And for this reason every effort is made to fulfill the desires associated with marriage and childbearing. However, childhood and pregnancy are two times when the individual is especially vulnerable and the possibility of an untimely death the greatest. Thus, it would seem that gratification of all wants would be an attempt to enhance the likelihood of release in the event of death and, conversely, to preclude the possibility of the self becoming a *bhut*.

Sorcery (*tuk*) also represents an example of the destructive consequences of frustrated desire. For example, there is a common belief that the childless woman's longing for a child may motivate her to bewitch another's child. Her desires are so strong that any indication of her attraction to a child arouses the fear that she may unintentionally cast an ''evil eye'' on the child. Generally, *tuk* is the result of envy and jealousy, where the presense of the other person is a reminder of what the sorcerer himself/herself lacks. The mother of an unsuccessful student might perform *tuk* on her son's more intelligent classmate. The jilted lover might bewitch the husband of his former lover. Or, the new bride might be the object of jealousy from almost anyone in her new household. Thus, *tuk* is the result of deprivation and the frustration of one's desires.

The Work of G. S. Bose

One of the things that struck me as I began to understand the pervasiveness of this theme of frustration is that it is quite reminiscent of Freud's theories of anxiety, repression, and mental disorder. It is not surprising, then, to find that psychoanalytic theory has attracted considerable attention in Bengal. The Indian Psychoanalytic Society has its national headquarters in Calcutta, and in 1976 fourteen of the thirty-nine qualified analysts resided there. It has established an in-patient facility (Lumbini Park Mental Hospital), an out-patient clinic (G. S. Bose Clinic) and two journals (*Samiksa* and *Chitta*). The English journal *Samiksa* began publication in 1947, three years before the Indian Psychiatric Association began publication of its journal. The Indian Psychoanalytic Institute has been training analysts since 1930, whereas Calcutta University established the Diploma of Psychological Medicine only in 1959.

Since the prestige of psychoanalysis in Bengal can be attributed to the dynamic and charismatic personality of Girindrasekhar Bose, I want to examine his theory and its link with this theme of frustrated desire. Born in 1887, G. S. Bose received degrees in both medicine and psychology. In 1929, Bose became the Head of the Department of Psychology at Calcutta University and remained in that position for twenty years. It appears that Bose may have become familiar with Freud's work as early as 1909, and in 1921, he and Freud began a correspondence that was to last for sixteen years (See Ramana 1964).

The main features of Bose's work are clear in his ''theory of opposite wish.'' In this theory, Bose postulates that every wish is accompanied by its opposite. A wish, according to Bose (1966: 69), is ''a peculiar psychic process conscious or unconscious which precedes or accompanies the tendency of the organism in its effort to change the environment so as to have an adjustment different from the existing one.'' Bose argues that in order for the individual to formulate a wish, he must "have some sort of appreciation of the object" (1966: 71). This appreciation of and identification with the object, required in order to formulate a wish at all, necessitates that the individual must concomitantly formulate the opposite wish. "Every wish that arises in consciousness is accompanied by its opposite which remains in the unconscious" (1966: 82). Thus, an active wish is accompanied by a passive wish. The wish to strike is accompanied by the wish to be struck; the wish to love triggers the wish to be loved. For unless the individual understands what is implied by being struck or being loved through identification, he cannot desire to strike or to love. Wishes, then, for Bose, always exist as opposing pairs and each pair consists of an active wish and a passive wish. Since both wishes cannot be satisfied simultaneously, one of them will become repressed.

Thus, Bose used the term "wish" as comparable to Freud's id. While both of these are seen as motivational and energizing factors of the personality, there are two crucial differences. First, wish, as opposed to the id, is not instinctual; the content varies depending on the state of the individual and the particular relation to the environment. That wishes occur as an opposing pair is a logical "necessity," not a physiological one. Secondly, the motivational force of the wish is directed towards instrumental action, that is, towards achieving a changed adaptation to the environment. While it is certainly clear that the satisfaction of id drives also requires environmental response, the focus is more expressive than instrumental.

In Bose's work, repression seems to be more dependent on environmental frustration of wishes than is Freud's concept of repression. Bose (1966: 85) argues that "repeated compulsory satisfaction of one of the wishes of a pair to the neglect of the other owing to one-sided environmental influences is responsible for bringing about a repression of the latter wish." For Freud, suppression only becomes repression when the superego introjects the moral principles of the surrounding society, thus prohibiting even conscious awareness of id desires. Bose, however, saw the superego as the product of repression ("the opposite counterparts of the oedipus tendencies") and believed that his theory "will render the conception of superego unnecessary" (1960: 90). Freudian theory postulates a dynamic tension and conflict between the individual and the society which is lacking in Bose's work. By eliminating the superego as prior to repression and by linking the opposite wishes logically, Bose views the source of repression as residing either within the contradictory nature of wishes or within the environment.

From the previous discussion, the influence of the psychological assumptions from Bose's cultural environment is also clear. Indeed, it would seem that Bose may have found Freud's work congenial because it tended to reflect psychological conceptions already prevalent in Bengali culture. Bose's work could be said to represent a Freudian interpretation of themes that are recurrent both in the classical Sanskritic literature and in the cultural milieu of his own society. The id, as the motivational energy, is already recognizably similar to *kama* and *rajas*. By transforming the Freudian id into "wish," Bose is able to assimilate conceptions which are evident in his own cultural heritage. First, wish becomes the instrumental means of relating to the environment. Secondly, with the "theory of opposite wish," Bose asserts the destructive potential of wish, a theme found in both the Sanskrit literature and the ethnographic data. In both Hindu philosophy and Bose's psychoanalysis, it is the nature of man's desires which obstruct self-realization. From this perspective, Bose's work, as a study of "wish," can be seen to follow in the tradition of enquiring into the nature of *kama*, passion.

Desire in Bengali Ethnopsychology

This survey of the role of passion in Bengali ethnopsychology reveals the fundamental belief in the destructive capabilities of desire and passion. Two themes can be extracted. On the one hand, ethnographic evidence indicates that unsatisfied desires are believed to produce deleterious results and that a prerequisite for physical and psychological health is the gratification of desire. On the other hand, following the Sanskritic tradition, passion hinders liberation and thus a prerequisite of salvation is freedom from passion. On first inspection, the two themes do seem contradictory. While the first argues for the expression and fulfillment of desires, the second encourages the subjugation of desire and its elimination as a prelude to final release. However, I want now to examine how these two themes can be integrated into a common framework and to demonstrate the position of madness within that framework.

The ideal state of passionlessness does not refer to the suppression of desire but rather to the emancipation from desire. Thus, freedom from passion and the satisfaction of passion are both in opposition to a state of thwarted desire. Or, conversely, frustration can be avoided either by the satisfaction of desires or by the elimination of desire altogether. In this sense, the two themes simply provide two different alternatives to a culturally recognized malignant state. To use a metaphor which is particularly apt in the Indian context where passion is identified with heat, a state of "firelessness" can be achieved through extinguishing the fire (*i.e.*, gratification) or through controling the conditions which cause a fire (*i.e.*, self-control, detachment). My argument is that each alternative is appropriate for certain people in certain situations according to *sva-dharma*, their own specific moral code of conduct.

It is recognized that the task of learning to be free of passion is a gradual process. According to Hindu thought, the life cycle of the individual can be devided into four states (*asrama*)—apprenticeship, householder, hermit, and sage. While the earlier stages of life prepare the individual for release, it is only in the last stage when the individual is expected to gain control over his desires as a means to attain *moksha*. Thus, the Sanskrit doctrine of freedom from passion is applicable only to the individual within the last stage of life. Furthermore, as an intermediary stage on the way to ultimate emancipation, the fulfillment of desire is permitted and may actually facilitate ultimate renunciation. The implication is that attachment to the world may be strengthened when desires are frustrated.

Moreover, the determination of one's proper *sva-dharma* (personal duty) is not only dependent on *asrama* (stage of life), but also relative to one's other attributes (Kakar 1968). Thus, the *dharma* of a child or woman is considered different from that of a man in any of the stages of life. Childhood is not included in the *asramas*, and apprenticeship begins with a boy's "second birth" at the time of receiving the sacred thread at age 12 or 13. Until that time, the child does not possess the reason or intellect (i.e., the *guna*, attributes) required to begin the road to salvation. Similarly, the stages of life are not relevant to women. By virtue of the *guna* associated with femininity, "their true function was marriage and the care of their menfolk and children" (Basham 1959: 178). It would appear that the very nature (*guna*) of women and children negate the expectation to refrain from the expression and satisfaction of passion. And indeed, as we saw, it is just in the case of women and children that the cultural rule about not frustrating desires is most evident.

Thus, the two themes that I identified can be integrated by recognizing that the philosophico-religious directive to be free from passion is specific for a man at the stage of renunciation. For others, their inherent *guna* and the undeveloped state of their spirituality precludes emancipation from passion. Desire and its expression, if not valued, are at least to be expected. And since such persons are not able to control their passions, it is best that they be gratified. Figure 1 illustrates this relationship between the three states of desire. As alternatives to a negative and destructive state of frustrated desire, both gratification of desire and freedom from desire are acceptable, although passionlessness is the ideally preferred alternative. But given the very nature of children, women, and the spiritually immature, the gratification of desire is advantageous in the face of the detrimental, negative consequences of unfulfilled passion.

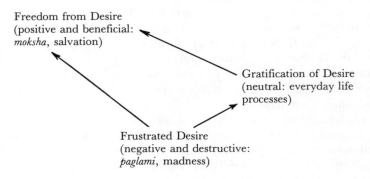

Freedom from Desire
(positive and beneficial:
moksha, salvation)

Gratification of Desire
(neutral: everyday life
processes)

Frustrated Desire
(negative and destructive:
paglami, madness)

Fig. 1. Desire in Bengali Ethnopsychology

Within this scheme, the position of *paglami* as deviance is clear. It is the direct result of frustrated desire—be it the "shock" of *mathar golmal* (head malfunctioning), the envy of *tuk* (sorcery), or the early death of *bhut bhɔr* (ghost possession). Madness or *paglami* becomes the concrete expression of the destructive and pernicious consequences of frustrated desire. Thus, as the deviance associated with ungratified desire *paglami* stands in juxtaposition to the everyday, neutral state of the satisfaction of desire and testifies to the harmful effects of frustrated desire. As a malignant state of human existence, *paglami* is a category of deviance which informs Bengalis of a basic human need—the need to avoid frustration and to obtain the satisfaction of one's wants and desire.

Furthermore, *paglami* testifies to the vulnerability of human beings in the face of the potent nature of their desires. So long as individuals rely on the gratification of passion to protect them from the destructive potential of their own emotions, they are dependent on the whims of an environment which can prevent such gratification. And, thus, *paglami* is a continual possibility: to quote again from the Gita, "craving (unfulfilled) leads to anger, and anger to confusion; confusion makes for unreasonableness and that results in madness, which is the road to destruction." It is in this sense that *paglami* represents an antithetical state from which the very meaning of salvation (*moksha*) is derived. By highlighting the very tentative and precarious relationship between human beings and their existential situation, *paglami* also indicates the solution to that human dilemma. To be mad is to be overwhelmed by one's emotions; to have attained salvation is to be released not only from one's desires but also from the vulnerability connected with the dependence on environmental gratification of desires.

REFERENCES

Ananda Bazar Patrika
    1975   Calcutta. August 4.
BECKER, Howard S.
    1963   *Outsiders: Studies in the Sociology of Deviance.* New York: The Free Press.
BHATTACHARYYA, Deborah P.
    1977   "Madness as Entropy: A Bengali View." Paper presented at the Bengal Studies
           Conference, Chicago, 1977.
BOSE, Girindrasekhar
    1966   *A New Theory of Mental Life.* Calcutta: Indian Psychoanalytic Association.
BRAR, H. S.
    1970   "Yoga and Psychoanalysis." *British Journal of Psychiatry* 16:201-206.
CARSTAIRS, G. Morris
    1956   "*Hinjra* and *Jiryan*: Two Derivatives of Hindu Attitudes to Sexuality. *British Journal
           of Medical Psychology* 29: 128-138.
    1957   *The Twice Born: A Study of a Community of High Caste Hindus.* London: The Hogarth
           Press.
COSTER, Geraldine
    1934   *Yoga and Western Psychiatry: A Comparison.* London: Oxford University Press.
DEBARY, William Theodore
    1958   *Sources of Indian Tradition.* Vol. 1. New York: Columbia University Press.
DESHMUKH, D. R.
    1972   "Experiments in the management of Psychological Disorders with Yoga." *Journal of
           the Yoga Institute* 18(5): 80-83.

ERIKSON, Kai
   1966   *Wayward Puritans: A Study in the Sociology of Deviance*. New York: John Wiley.
GOYECHE, R.
   1972   "Yoga as Psychotherapy." *Journal of the Yoga Institute* 18(1): 4-7.
JACOBS, Hans
   1961   *Western Psychotherapy and Hindu Sadhana: A Contribution to Comparative Studies in Psychology and Metaphysics*. London: George ALLAN.
JOSHI, H. M.
   1964   "Indian Approach to Psychology." *Darshana International* 4(2): 58-69.
KAKAR, Sudhir
   1968   "The Human Life Cycle: The Traditional Hindu View and the Psychology of Erik Erikson." *Philosophy East and West* 18: 127-136.
   1978   *The Inner World: A Psychoanalytic Study of Childhood and Society in India*. Delhi: Oxford University Press.
MASSON, J. Moussareff
   1974   "Sex and Yoga: Psychoanalysis and the Indian Religious Experience." *Journal of Indian Philosophy* 2: 307-320.
MURPHY, Gardner and Lois B. MURPHY (eds.)
   1968   *Asian Psychology*. New York: Basic Books.
OBEYESEKERE, Gananath
   1976   "The Impact of Ayurvedic Ideas on the Culture and the Individual in Sri Lanka." *In* Charles Leslie (ed.), *Asian Medical Systems*. Berkeley: University of California Press. Pp. 210-226.
PAL, Kumar
   1971   "Comparison of Yoga and Psychoanalysis." *Darshana International* 2(1): 49-67.
RAMANA, C. V.
   1964   "On the Early History and Development of Psychoanalysis in India." *American Psychoanalytic Association Journal* 12: 110-134.
RAO, S. K. Ramachandra
   1962   *Development of Psychological Thought in India*. Mysore: Kavyalaya Publishers.
SPRATT, Philip
   1966   *Hindu Culture and Personality: A Psychoanalytic Study*. Bombay: Manaktalas.
SURYA, N. C.
   1969   "Ego Structure in the Hindu Joint Family: Some Considerations." *In* William Caudill and Tsung-yi Lin (eds.), *Mental Health Research in Asia and the Pacific*. Honolulu: East-West Center Press. Pp. 381-392.
VAHIA, N. S.
   1969   "A Therapy Based upon Some Concepts Prevalent in India." *Indian Journal of Psychiatry* 2(1-2): 7-14.
VAHIA, N. S. et al
   1966   "Some Ancient Indian Concepts in the Treatment of Psychiatric Disorders." *British Journal of Psychiatry* 112: 1089-1096.
   1972   "A Deconditioning Therapy Based upon Concepts of Patanjali." *International Journal of Social Psychiatry* 18(1): 61-68.
   1973a "Further Experience with the Therapy Based upon Concepts of Patanjali in the Treatment of Psychiatric Disorders." *Indian Journal of Psychiatry* 15(1): 32-37.
   1973b "Psychophysiologic Therapy Based on the Concepts of Patanjali." *American Journal of Psychotherapy* 27(4): 557-565.

Concepts of Person and Situation in North Indian Counseling

The Case of Astrology

JUDY F. PUGH *

University of British Columbia, Vancouver, Canada

ASTROLOGERS FORM A VITAL SOURCE of aid and advice for dealing with the dilemmas and difficulties of everyday life in India. They counsel clients on a wide range of problems, including family conflicts, problems of education and occupation, financial troubles, political ambition, and various kinds of physical and psychological ailments. In the course of a typical advisory session, the client discusses his problem with the astrologer, who uses the interpretation of horoscopes, palms, divinatory texts, and other devices to focus the discussion; the astrologer identifies planetary influences and sometimes other factors which have contributed to the development of the client's present set of circumstances; and he recommends one or more remedies, including charms, rings, worship, almsgiving, herbal decoctions, and other kinds of ameliorative behavior. Astrological consultation, then, involves the use of ancient, textually mediated traditions to deal with a broad spectrum of seemingly heterogeneous ailments, conflicts, and dilemmas, providing an important source of counseling for Indians of all social and economic levels.

The questions of how theory and practice are articulated in astrological counseling, and how order is constituted in the diagnosis and treatment of a disparate array of problems, are fundamental to an understanding of astrology as a therapeutic system. The most elucidating answers to these questions may derive from a phenomenological perspective which aims to understand the symbolic organization of the astrological counseling process and its representations of everyday life. In the present paper I suggest that concepts of the person constitute a central part of this symbolic organization, and I explore ways in which these concepts inform the discourse on experience which is embedded in the counseling process. It is, after all, the person whose destiny, whose *karma* or *qismat*, is reflected in the stars and whose circumstances are considered to show

* *Acknowledgments.* This paper is based on fieldwork carried out in Banaras from January 1975 to June 1976. I am indebted to the Social Science Research Council for a dissertation research fellowship which generously supported my work. I would also like to thank McKim Marriott, Ralph Nicholas, and Victor Turner for their comments on earlier versions of my work on concepts of the person, particularly my doctoral dissertation.

certain broadly determinate patterns. Conceptually congruent notions of the person appear to be expressed in astrological classifications and in divinatory dialogues between astrologer and client, as well as in informally parlanced routines of everyday life, thus constituting a fundamental aspect of the cultural system through which Indians perceive and experience basic life-problems.

The debate between Dumont and Marriott on the question of the individual and the nature of the person in South Asian culture and society (see Dumont 1970; Marriott and Inden 1972; Marriott 1976) has served to point up ways in which these notions vary between Western and Indian ideological systems. Other studies in the Asian context (for instance, Chang 1977; Geertz 1973; Ortner 1978; Rosaldo 1980) also report a differently constructed notion of personhood than that which prevails in Western social thought. And medical anthropology now recognizes the importance of including theories of the person in analyses of illness and healing (see Lewis 1975: 6; Fortes 1976; Janzen 1978: 157-193; Comaroff 1980). The task here, as in social anthropology and social thought more generally, is to describe indigenous conceptual systems in such a way as to be able to develop from these descriptions a set of culturally-grounded analytic perspectives, including perspectives on the experience of illness and healing. In view of this task, it is essential not to place *a priori* limits on the notions of personhood which we set out to explore. This means, for instance, that description should not be arbitrarily restricted to the biological or spiritual make-up of the person (cf. Fortes 1976; Lewis 1976), but rather that the possibility should be admitted that other cultural systems may "draw the effective boundary of the person differently, more expansively, than classical Western medicine, philosophy, and religion" (Janzen 1978: 189).

Astrological counseling has a different centerpoint than therapeutic systems concerned specifically with sickness: it focuses instead on the client's problems or problematic situations. This focus involves a total socioexistential manifold in which sickness figures as one among several major sources of difficulty. The fact of this socioexistential focus reinforces the importance of setting a broad descriptive compass for the study of person-concepts, while it also suggests that certain theoretical constructs in the field of medical anthropology—specifically those constructs hinged on a presumption of the ontological primacy of disease—should be reexamined in terms of their utility for the cross-cultural analysis of counseling processes. Significantly, the analysis of the broad compass of problems taken up in astrological counseling requires an interpretive perspective whose terms and ultimate theoretical aims do not derive from nor point back to the phenomenon of sickness but rather work from and toward problematic experiences in the life of the person.

The description and analysis of problematic experiences in the person's life can be culturally sensitized not only by examining concepts of the person but also (and coordinately) by looking at indigenous concepts of the situation and their articulation with theories of the person. The notion of "situation" has been an important analytic construct in Western social thought (see Parsons 1951: 4-23; Schutz 1967: 163-172; McHugh 1968: 7-20; Goffman 1974:

1-20). In this tradition, "situation" refers primarily to an interactional arena or frame in which both verbal and non-verbal behavioral processes create and enact an intersubjectively articulated set of rules and meanings. This concept of "situation" emphasizes concrete behavioral settings and tends to overlook the availability of other meanings of "situation" which might capture more fully the subjective worlds in which people live. Meanings of "situation" such as "circumstances," "condition," and "case" inform everyday life and commonplace English usage, and similar concepts are expressed in Indian society in everyday speech and also figure in the presentation and analysis of problems in the context of divinatory counseling.[1] These meanings refer less to a concrete behavioral setting and more to a subjectively perceived state of affairs—a network of meaning which links together a variegated array of events, persons, and experiences.

The present paper deals, then, with the articulation between concepts of the person and concepts of the situation which underlies the therapeutic discourse of astrological counseling. This methodological orientation facilitates the description of person and situation as a phenomenologically unified field of experience, thus providing an alternative to ontologically discontinuous methods for the study of the person in the context of healing. It is common in medical anthropology that "mind" and "body" are treated primarily as indigenous concepts, while "family" and "community" are discussed as "real" groups.[2] Discontinuous concatenations of positivistic and interpretive methodologies are also reflected in a distinction between "person" as an indigenous conceptual entity and "situation" as a concrete context of interaction, and alternately, in an understanding of the person's affective life as constituting an experiential phenomenon and his "social" existence as involving concrete situational contexts.[3]

The intriguing question is how do indigenous concepts of the person order (and thereby constrain) the kinds of therapeutic discourse and the forms of treatment which are perceived as meaningful in a particular cultural or clinical setting.[4] One way to explore this ordering process is to examine the images of problematic situations which are constructed in the interaction between the astrologer or diviner and his client. This means that it is necessary to construe "culture" far more broadly than do studies in which the belief system which legitimates divinatory counseling is described primarily in terms of a few key "cosmological" notions, such as "fate" or "witchcraft."

From this perspective, it is also necessary to question whether we can invoke the operation of psychological mechanisms (such as anxiety-reduction, catharsis, transference, placebo effect, etc.) in the divinatory context without the support of a full description of the subtle representations of person and experience which inform the divinatory inquire.[5] One of the problems here is that the meaningfulness of the content of the constructive and projective activity in divinatory interactions usually receives less descriptive and analytic attention than does the functional role of divination in reducing anxiety and restoring confidence. This emphasis reflects too strong a psychiatric orientation to

divination as "the management of anxiety" and too undeveloped an interpretive sensitivity to divination as "the management of meaning."[6] These differences in theoretical perspective point up broad and complex issues in the
study of the organization and effectiveness of counseling processes cross-
culturally, and in the present essay I present a preliminary statement on the
structure of these processes in the context of astrological therapy.[7]

The Hindu and Muslim communities of the city of Banaras[8] provide the
ethnographic setting for my discussion of astrological counseling and the concepts of person and situation which it articulates. Astrology has a very lengthy
history in both Hinduism and Islam, and these two astrological traditions are
evident today in the work of the city's Hindu astrologers (*jyotishī*) and also in
the skills of some of its Muslim learned men (*maulvī*) who include astrology in
their diagnostic procedures.[9] The field of astrological and divinatory therapy,
although it receives differently valued emphases in the lives of Hindus and
Muslims, nonetheless forms an area of shared understandings: Hindus may
consult Muslim learned men, and Muslims may consult Hindu astrologers and
diviners, thus sustaining and reflecting a discourse which shows important in-
tercommunity continuities in the conceptualization of problematic life-
experiences and their treatment.

Aspects of the Person[10]

Astrology schematizes four mutually coincident aspects of the person: a
physical (*shārīrik*) aspect, a psychological (*mānsik*) aspect, and two social aspects
of familial (*pārivārik*) and community (*sāmājik*) relationships. Let me first
describe each of these four aspects of the person and then discuss ways in which
these concepts inform the astrological analysis of the client's circumstances and
the prescription of ameliorative remedies.

The body

The body (*sharīr, badan*) is a key conceptual aspect of the person, and
astrology schematizes important features of the body. The somatic systems
which astrology outlines include the gross limbic anatomy, the tissues, the
humors, the elements, and the qualitative attributes of hotness/coldness and
moistness/dryness. These systems and their associations with constellations
and planets are shown in Table 1.

In both Hindu and Islamic astrology the sectors (*ang*) of the gross anatomy
are linked with the constellations and planets. In the linkage between constellations and parts of the body, the head is linked with Aries (the first
constellation), the face with the second constellation Taurus, and so on, covering the parts of the anatomy (arms, chest, stomach, waist, hips, genitals,
thighs, knees, calves, feet) and the progression of the constellations.

The constellations and planets are also linked with the tissues whose relations constitute the person's physiological processes. The most important of

Table 1

The Astrological Schematization of the Body

Constellation (Rāshi; Burj)	Planet (Graha; Sitārā)	Gross Anatomy (Ang)	Tissue (Dhātu; 'Aza)
Aries	Mars	Head (Sir)	Stomach (Peṭ) Flesh (Māns, Gosht) Marrow (Gūdā, Majjā) Nose (Nāk)
Taurus	Venus	Face (Mukh)	Semen (Shukra) Womb (Garbha) Kidney (Gurdā)
Gemini	Mercury	Arms (Bāhu)	Brain (Dimāg) Tongue (Zabān) Skin (Tvachā, Khāl)
Cancer	Moon	Chest (Chhātī)	Eye (Ānkh) Breast (Stan) Lungs (Phephṛā) Blood (Rakta, Khūn)
Leo	Sun	Stomach (Peṭ)	Ear (Kān) Bones (Haḍḍi) Heart (Hṛday, Dil)
Virgo	Mercury	Waist (Kamar)	Brain (Dimāg) Tongue (Zabān) Skin (Tvachā, Khāl)
Libra	Venus	Hips (Nitamb)	Semen (Shukra) Womb (Garbha) Kidney (Gurdā)
Scorpio	Mars	Genitals (Linga)	Nose (Nāk) Stomach (Peṭ) Flesh (Mans, Gosht) Marrow (Gūdā, Majjā)
Sagittarius	Jupiter	Thigh (Janghā)	Fat (Charbī) Liver (Jigar) Intestine (Antṛī)
Capricorn	Saturn	Knees (Ghuṭnā)	Hair (Bāl) Ligaments (Snāyu)
Aquarius	Saturn	Calves (Piṇḍlī)	Hair (Bāl) Ligaments (Snāyu)
Pisces	Jupiter	Feet (Pair)	Fat (Charbī) Liver (Jigar) Intestine (Antṛī)

these tissues include the brain, tongue, hair, skin, flesh, ligaments, heart, lungs, breast, circulatory system, stomach, fat, liver, kidneys, sexual fluids, womb, intestines, and bones. Hindu thought gives particular emphasis to seven of these "constituent substances": bone, blood, flesh, fat, ligaments, skin, and semen. These substances are constantly regenerated through the metabolism of foods.

Table 1—Continued

Humor (Hindu System) (*Tridosha*)	Humor (Islamic System) (*Akhlāt*)	Element (*Bhūta*; '*Anāsar*)	Hot/Cold (*Garam/ Thanda*)	Wet/Dry (*Nam/Sūkh*) (*Tar/Khushk*)
Bile (*Pitta*)	Yellow bile (*Safrā*)	Fire (*Agni*; *Ātish*)	Hot	Dry
Wind (*Vāyu*)	Black bile (*Saudā*)	Earth (*Prithvī*; *Khāk*)	Cold	Wet
All 3 (*Sam*)	Blood (*Khūn*)	Air (*Vāyu*; *Bād*)	Hot	Wet
Phlegm (*Kaf*)	Phlegm (*Balgam*)	Water (*Jal*; *Āb*)	Cold	Wet
Bile (*Pitta*)	Yellow bile (*Safrā*)	Fire (*Agni*; *Ātish*)	Hot	Dry
Wind (*Vāyu*)	Black bile (*Saudā*)	Earth (*Prithvī*; *Khāk*)	Cold	Dry
All 3 (*Sam*)	Blood (*Khūn*)	Air (*Vāyu*; *Bād*)	Hot	Wet
Phlegm (*Kaf*)	Phlegm (*Balgam*)	Water (*Jal*; *Āb*)	Cold	Wet
Bile (*Pitta*)	Yellow bile (*Safrā*)	Fire (*Agni*; *Ātish*)	Hot	Dry
Wind (*Vāyu*)	Black bile (*Saudā*)	Earth (*Prithvī*; *Khāk*)	Cold	Dry
All 3 (*Sam*)	Blood (*Khūn*)	Air (*Vāyu*; *Bād*)	Hot	Wet
Phlegm (*Kaf*)	Phlegm (*Balgam*)	Water (*Jal*; *Āb*)	Cold	Wet

The system of humors (*tridosha, akhlāt*) is also linked with the celestial realm. Hindu astrology delimits a system of three humors: wind (*vāyu*), phlegm (*shleshmā, kaf*), and bile (*pitta*). Islamic astrology describes a system of four humors: blood (*khūn*), phlegm (*balgam*), black bile (*saudā*), and yellow bile (*safrā*).

The humoral system is linked to a system of base elements (*bhūta, 'anāsar*). These elements constitute the protean ground of both the heavens and the earth. Hindu astrology recognizes five elements: ether (*ākāsha*), air (*vāyu*), fire (*agni*), earth (*prithvī*), and water (*jal*). Islamic astrology recognizes four elements: air (*bād*), fire (*ātish*), water (*āb*), and earth (*khāk*). As Table 1 indicates, these elements are manifested in the humors: in the Hindu system, fire is manifested in bile, water in phlegm, earth in wind, and air in all three humors; in the Islamic system, fire is manifested in yellow bile, earth in black bile, water in phlegm, and air in blood. The elements are also manifested in the qualitative attributes of hotness/coldness and moistness/dryness: fire is hot and dry, earth is cold and dry, air is hot and wet, and water is cold and wet.

These systems constitute a notion of the body which is recognized in learned and popular medical theory in North India. Special emphasis is given in indigenous medical theory to the system of humors and the qualities of hot/cold and moist/dry. The balances and imbalances in these systems are considered to underlie the development of physical disorders. The congruence of the heavenly bodies with these balances is recognized in the indigenous systems of Ayurveda and Yunani.

Such an astrological schematization of the body is compatible with many categories of functional and pathogenic illnesses recognized in Western medicine. These include such common complaints as colds and other respiratory ailments, skin eruptions, various aches and pains, fevers, dizziness, and weakness, as well as such major diseases as tuberculosis, malaria, heart disease, kidney disease, cancer, smallpox, cholera, and others. Links between the planets and various parts of the body provide bases for assessing planetary influence on particular ailments. For example, as Table 1 shows, the moon is linked with the blood, and since malaria is considered to be a disease of the blood, the moon is believed to influence and indicate the person's particular susceptibility to malaria; smallpox, as an affliction of the skin, is especially influenced by Mercury; heart disease is influenced by the sun, and so on. In this way astrologers may diagnose and predict a wide array of infections, injuries, and malfunctions.

According to astrology the combinations of features of these somatic systems are given to each person at the time of birth. The person begins life with a template whose particular organization is reflected in the configurations of the heavens at the time and place of his birth.[11] This template guides the person's physical development, as well as the development of his other aspects, and the particular strengths and weaknesses which it encodes influence the person's good health (*svasthya, tandurustī*) or ill health (*rog, bīmārī*) during the entire course of his life. Astrology, along with learned and popular biological understandings, recognizes that the person's health is affected not only by the planets and constellations, but also by such factors as climate, diet, mental condition, and interpersonal relations. The template with which the person begins life sets the specific pattern of health and disease to which he will be susceptible, and the strength of celestial powers together with the person's own actions determine the extent to which these susceptibilities will be realized.

The psyche

A second aspect of the person is conceived to be what we might translate as psyche or psychological character. North Indians commonly locate the rational, discriminative faculty in the intellect (*buddhi, dimāg*), the affective, expressive faculty in the heart-mind (*man, hriday, dil*), and the most enduring faculty in the subtle body or soul (*ātma, rūḥ*). Astrology describes psychological traits within the context of a matrix of seven psychic faculties (Table 2). These include: the soul (*ātma, rūḥ*); the heart-mind (*man, hriday, dil*); the intellect (*buddhi, dimāg*) and the voice (*vānī, āwāz*); strength (*bal*); semen (*shukra, vīrya*); happiness (*sukh, khushī*); and sadness (*dukh*).

Table 2

The Planetary Schematization of Psychological
Faculties and Characteristics

Planet	Faculties	Characteristics	Affects
Sun (*Sūrya*; *Shams*)	(1) Soul (*Ātma*; *Rūḥ*)	Pre-eminence Authoritativeness Religiousness	Confidence Self-Assurance
Moon (*Chandra*; *Qamar*)	(2) Heart-Mind (*Man*, *hṛday*; *dil*)	Affectionateness Expressiveness	Love Sensitivity
Mars (*Mangal*; *Marīkh*)	(3) Strength (*Bal*)	Powerfulness Aggressiveness	Anger Conflict
Mercury (*Budh*; *'Atarad*)	(4) Intellect (*Buddhi*; *Dimāg*) & Voice (*Vānī*; *Āwāz*)	Intellectualness Articulateness	Nervousness
Jupiter (*Bṛihaspati, Guru*; *Mushterī*)	(4) Intellect (*Buddhi*; *Dimāg*) (5) Happiness (*Sukh*; *Khushī*)	Intellectualness Wisdom Happiness	Happiness
Venus (*Shukra*; *Zohrā*)	(6) Semen (*Shukra*, *Vīrya*)	Sexualness	Passion
Saturn (*Shani*; *Zoḥal*)	(7) Sadness (*Dukh*)	Sadness	Sadness Fear

Table 3

The Planetary Schematization of
"Qualitative Strands" (Guṇa)

Sun	Moon	Mars	Mercury	Venus	Jupiter	Saturn
Sattva	Sattva	Tamas	Rajas	Rajas	Sattva	Tamas

The seven psychic faculties of the person which astrology schematizes assume particular values for each person, and together these organize his characteristic psychology. Some typifications refer to these psychological faculties, so that the person is typified according to particuar values of pre-eminence and authoritativeness, affectionateness, sexualness, powerfulness, wisdom, sadness, happiness, intellectualness, and articulateness. Other typifications reflect the view that physical processes affect the temperament. For instance, the person may be characterized as "bile natured" (*pitta prakṛiti*), "of phlegmatic temperament" (*kaf svabhāva*), or "fiery tempered" (*agni svabhāva*), with the references indicating actual influences of particular imbalances in the person's somatic systems on his characteristic psychological nature.

The affective or expressive faculty is given special elaboration in astrological classifications and in the use of these categories in the advisory session. In this scheme, the Sun indicates confidence or self-assurance, the Moon indicates love and sensitivity, Mars anger and conflict, Mercury nervousness, Venus passion, Jupiter happiness, and Saturn sadness and fear. These general categories of affect can also accommodate a range of more specific affects, some of which, such as anxiety, can be indicated by more than one planet. These basic forms of affective expression are understood to form part of the person's experiential existence, which means that they are intimately implicated in all sorts of problematic situations which constitute the ordinary course of life.

The Hindu view of the psyche also stresses a system of "strands" or attributes" (*guṇa*) which are described in Hindu philosophy and also comprehended in popular understandings. These strands or attributes are not substances in themselves, but variously combine to characterize all substances and actions. They include goodness or lightness (*sattva*), passion (*rajas*), and darkness and inertia (*tamas*). All three of these qualities constantly interact to affect the person's psychical and interpersonal character, and the planets are considerered to influence the proportionality among them (Table 3). Hindu characterizations of the person's temperament also employ these qualities: a person with an active, benevolent nature is described as "light natured" or "good tempered" (*sāttvik guṇa svabhāva*); a person with a volatile nature is described as "passion tempered" (*rajasik guṇa svabhāva*); a person with a slothful nature is described as "lazy tempered" (*rajāsik guṇa svabhāva*).

In the North Indian view the person is believed to be marked by his gross bodily characteristics and also by an enduring set of these subtler psychic characteristics. Together they constitute his personal nature or temperament (*svabhāva, mizāj*). The particular characteristics of the person's psychical faculties are believed to be established, like those of his physical body, at the time his life begins.

Astrology also recognizes that the person's temperament, like his body, is influenced not only by the planets and stars but also by climate, diet, and interpersonal relations. Astrology works on the assumption of a close articulation between the person's psyche and his body, so that any influences on the psyche are also influences on the body and on social relationships and vice versa.

Family and community relationships

The person is also constituted by his familial (*pārivārik*) and community (*sāmājik*) relationships. The family (*parivār, khāndān*) is a primordial human environment whose members are joined through shared bodily substance and shared codes for conduct (Marriott and Inden 1972; Inden and Nicholas 1977). Astrology schematizes categories of kinsmen and their association with planetary bodies (Table 4). These include father, mother, older brother, younger brother, sister, husband, wife, mother's brother, daughter, son, grandson, paternal grandfather, and maternal grandfather.

Table 4

The Planetary Schematization of Kinsmen

Planet	Kinsman
Sun (*Sūrya*; *Shams*)	Father (*Pitā*; *Wālid*)
Moon (*Chandra*; *Qamar*)	Mother (*Mātā*; *Mā*)
Mars (*Mangal*; *Marīkh*)	Brother (*Bhāī*) Sister (*Bahin*)
Mercury (*Budh*; *'Atarad*)	Mother's brother (*Māmā*)
Jupiter (*Bṛihaspati, Guru*; *Mushterī*)	Son (*Beṭā, Putra, Laṛkā*) Daughter (*Beṭī, Putrī, Laṛkī*) Grandson (*Potā*) Granddaughter (*Potī*)
Venus (*Shukra*; *Zohrā*)	Husband (*Pati*; *Shauhar*) Wife (*Patnī*; *Bīwī*)
Saturn (*Shani*; *Zoḥal*)	Paternal Grandfather (*Dādā*) Maternal Grandfather (*Nānā*)

Table 5

The Planetary Schematization of Fields of Activity
and Occupational Categories

Planet	Field of Activity	Occupational Category
Sun (*Sūrya*; *Shams*)	Government (*Sarkār*; *Ḥukūmat*)	King (*Rājā*; *Bādshāh*) Minister (*Mantrī*; *Vazīr*) Govt. worker (*Sarkārī naukar*)
	Medicine (*Chikitsā*; *Ṭibb*)	Doctor (*Ḍākṭar, Vaidya, Ḥakīm*)
Moon (*Chandra*; *Qamar*)	Medicine (*Chikitsā*; *Ṭibb*)	Doctor (*Ḍākṭar, Vaidya, Hakīm*)
	Agriculture (*Kṛishi*; *Khetī*)	Farmer (*Kisān*) Landlord (*Zamīndār*)
Mars (*Mangal*; *Marīkh*)	Military (*Senā*; *Fauj*)	Soldier (*Sainik*; *Sipāhī*)
Mercury (*Budh*; *'Atārad*)	Business (*Vyāpār*; *Saudāgarī*)	Merchant (*Vyāpārī*; *Saudāgar*)
Jupiter (*Brihaspati, Guru*; *Mushterī*)	Religion (*Dharma*; *Dīn*)	Priest (*Pujārī*; *Mullā*)
	Education (*Shikshā*; *Tālīm*)	Teacher (*Guru, Adhyāpak*; *Ustād*) Student (*Vidyārthī*; *Tālib*)
Venus (*Shukra*; *Zohrā*)	Art (*Kalā*; *Kārīgarī*)	Artist (*Kalākār*; *Kārīgar*)
Saturn (*Shani*; *Zoḥal*)	Crime (*Aprādh*; *Jurm*)	Thief (*Chor*)

These categories of kinsmen designate the person's central familial relationships. They indicate the relationships which are characteristically primary in the person's familial life, and because of the reciprocal nature of role definitions, they also designate the kin-categories which mark the person himself. These ties of kin relatedness are intrinsic to the conceptualization of the person in North Indian culture, and placement at the center of a collection of kinsmen is an essential feature of the person in astrological representations.

The person is also conceived to be naturally implicated in social relationships beyond the family. Astrology schematizes these interpersonal or community relationships by a set of primarily occupational categories (Table 5). Persons of these categories include: king, minister, and government worker, from the field of government; doctor and patient, from the field of medicine; farmer and landlord, from the field of agriculture; soldier, from the field of the military; merchant, customer, and partner, from the field of business; priest, from the field of religion; teacher and student, from the field of education; artist, from the field of art; and thief, from the field of crime.

The categories of the person's family and community relationships are considered to be mutually constituted along with those of his physical and psychical qualities. His interpersonal relationships are structured coincidentally with his mental and physical condition. Factors of harmony and discord in family and community relationships are conjoined with physical and psychological factors in the organization of the person's daily life.

Advisory Consultation

The astrological advisory session is used for several different kinds of purposes: (1) matching horoscopes for prospective marriage partners; (2) selecting an auspicious time for an important undertaking; (3) having a birth-horoscope cast; (4) getting a general assessment of one's current situation, along with a protective or remedial device such as a charm; (5) getting diagnosis and treatment for a specific problem. In the present context I am concerned with the last two activities—getting a general assessment of one's current situation and seeking diagnosis and treatment for a specific problem. The therapeutic interaction between astrologer and client is actually very similar in these two instances, since a client who asks for a general view of his situation is in fact usually concerned about several specific problems.

The advisory interaction between astrologer and client is organized around the divinatory dialogue. This dialogue incorporates the astrologer's interpretation of divinatory devices, such as horoscopes, palms, dice, and labeled tokens, and the verbal and non-verbal exchanges between astrologer and client. As therapeutic discourse this dialogue sustains a complex process of projective and constructive activity through which the astrologer uses the symbolic classifications of astrology to elicit, sharpen, enlarge, and confirm the client's account of his own situation. When the client consults an astrologer in order to get a general assessment of his current circumstances, it is usual for the astrologer to initiate the analysis and to provide a preliminary outline of his situation, which is then explored, modified, and perhaps expanded. When a client seeks advice on a specific problem, he usually mentions his main concerns to the astrologer at the outset, and then he and the astrologer use the divinatory dialogue in tandem with the astrologer's accompanying interpretation of any of several divinatory devices, in order to explore the specific details of the problem.

From the perspective of Indian astrological hermeneutics, the divinatory dialogue takes up the surface contours of everyday life and renders them meaningful in ways which do not depend on or theoretically invoke the operation of depth psychoanalytic processes. If this is so, then what does constitute the source of order and meaning in these divinatory interactions? How does astrological divination provide for the interpretation and treatment of the seemingly heterogeneous array of problems and concerns which North Indians bring for consultation? The highly subjective and ostensibly idiosyncratic nature of this enormous variety of situations might be considered to render them intransient to social scientific analysis. What I would like to show in the present section is that the underlying order which informs this variegated array of personal situations is provided by the concept of the person. As we have seen, the person is conceptualized in terms of four mutually coincident aspects of body, mind, and family and community relationships, and it is these four aspects which together constitute the underlying matrix from which specific experiential configurations are organized.

The category of "problem" or "problematic situation" provides the general framework for presenting and discussing complaints and dilemmas in the astrological context. The concept of the situation (*paristhiti, hālāt*) refers to a configuration of experiences (*anubhava, tajarbā*) which takes on particular relevance durig a given period of time. The person's situation is conceptualized as a set of circumstances or a field of experiences which prevails in his life during a given period of time.

Let me illustrate the articulation between concepts of the situation and concepts of the person by describing four different examples of situations analyzed in astrological advisory sessions in Banaras. I select these particular examples of situations because they indicate cultural and clinical continuities between Hindus and Muslims, because they show continuities across four different methods of astrological divination, and because they reveal parallels between relatively simple and relatively complex personal situations.

The first situation is one presented by a Muslim client to a Hindu roadside astrologer. The client outlines his situation as follows: "I am feeling anxiety because of my son's sickness and my wife's unhappiness." After this introductory statement, the astrologer examines the man's palm and tells him more about his situation—he has other children and they are well, this child will get better, and his wife will again be happy. He says that the cause of these difficulties has been the planet Mars and that this malevolent influence is now passing.

After further discussion of the situation, the astrologer recommends several remedies (*ilāj*): he tells the man to feed Muslim holy men and animals, and he gives him a small piece of wood to serve as a charm (*ta'wīz*) for providing protection against harmful influences. The astrologer adds that he can see that the man is already doing his prayers regularly, so that that source of aid is being looked after. These particular remedies—charitable acts, charms, and prayer—are intended both to protect against the influences of Mars and to enlist divine aid in the restoration of the situation as a whole—the restoration of the son's health and the removal of the wife's unhappiness and the man's anxiety.

This situation (Fig. 1) involves a particular set of circumstances with which the client is currently concerned. The man's anxiety (*chintā*) is linked with his son's sickness (*bīmārī*) and his wife's unhappiness (*dukh*), which is also related to the son's sickness. The situation conjoins categories of kinsmen (in the specificity of the kin-types "wife," "son," and "children") with categories of body (in the specificity of "sickness") and mind (in the specificity of "anxiety" and "unhappiness").

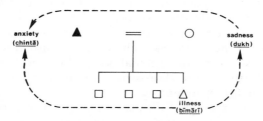

Fig. 1.—The client's situation

In view of the importance which many studies of divination attach to the naming of causal agents (see, for instance, Horton 1967; Jansen 1973) it is essential to note that here the identification of causal forces occurs as part of the process of situation construction. The conceptualization of the situation is essential to the delineation of the several levels of causation which appear to operate—the overarching influence of Mars (itself a manifestation of the workings of destiny) and the influence of the son's sickness on his parents' affective condition, or more accurately, the influence of the son's sickness on the mother's psychological condition and the influence of both of these factors on the father's psychological condition. In short, this structurally simple situation involves an experientially dense configuration of basic life-concerns.

A second example of a situation is provided by a Hindu client who discusses his political ambitions with a widely respected Brahman astrologer. This particular divinatory dialogue relies on a horoscope reading and involves a lengthy conversation between the astrologer and the client, with occasional comments and questions added by a friend accompanying the client. The client's situation is outlined as follows (Fig. 2):

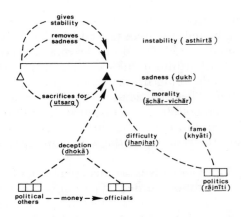

Fig. 2. The client's situation

His career fortunes have been in flux and he has been prone to sadness (depression?); he is aiming for political renown but is encountering difficulties; someone else has bribed election officials and they have deceived him; his younger brother has already made sacrifices for him and can serve as an important source of stability and happiness. These features are indicated in a general way by the positions of several constellations (Libra and Sagittarius) and the planets Saturn and Jupiter in the horoscope, and they receive added specificity and extension through the divinatory dialogue. The astrologer recommends, first, a topaz ring to augment positive planetary influences, specifically those of Jupiter, the planet associated with fame and preeminence; second, a schedule of astrologically timed decisions about when to stand for what elections; third a pattern of morally informed behavior.

A third example of a problematic situation is provided by a Hindu client's consultation with a Muslim learned man who uses dice (*ramal*) to identify planetary and other influences. In this case the client asks for a general assessment of his situation; the diviner asks him to throw the dice; and he then calculates the throw and checks the resulting ideogram in a text of prognosticatory indications. He then outlines the following set of circumstances: "You have a good income, but your expenditures are also sizeable. There is disappointment from going on a journey. You are angry with your wife. Some danger is coming up. Be clever. This Mars will fight. During this January which is just ending, you are spending your time in fighting, quarreling, and brawling (Fig. 3).

The client's situation is clearly marked by degenerative transformations in his sociofamilial relationships and the affective conditions which are complicit with them. Conflict is manifested in his anger with his wife and in his quarreling with unnamed other persons, and he is also suffering some disappointment. Economic troubles add to this picture of a precarious set of circumstances. The diviner associates these troubles with the planet Mars, which

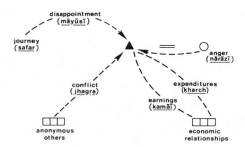

Fig. 3. The client's situation

is associated with conflict and anger, and with a longer cycle of Saturn, notorious for its destructive and baleful influences. Two kinds of remedies are recommended by the diviner—worship and the wearing of a sapphire to ward off Saturnian influences.

A fourth case shows a Muslim husband and wife consulting a Muslim learned man. Their presenting complaint is the woman's sickness. The *maulvi* asks the woman to select a token from a dish, and as he begins to question her, he makes several calculations on the basis of the markings on this token. While he is completing these calculations, he talks with the woman in order to lay out the disturbances which have marked her psychophysical condition for some six months—nervousness, insomnia, palpitations, gastrointestinal complaints, and weakness. During this discussion he announces that her sickness is caused by something evil which someone has done. The dialogue proceeds, and at the woman's instigation, the discussion turns to conflicts in her household. The source of these conflicts appears to be the activities of her husband's younger brother, who has lapsed into a pattern of irresponsible behavior toward the household. The dialogue proceeds to cover various aspects of this problem and to link it to the woman's debilitated condition. It is interesting that in this case the *maulvi* explicitly rules out malevolent planetary influence and focuses instead on human agency as the source of trouble. We see, then, that in this picture of the situation, the transformations in the woman's physical and mental condition from health to illness have developed in the context of changes in family relations from unity to discord and from fulfillment of responsibility to neglect of responsibility (Fig. 4).

In this case, the *maulvi* recommends several kinds of remedies—charms for the woman to wear and to keep in the house, an herbal decoction to drink (this particular decoction contains active ingredients which exert a sedative effect and soothe stomach and intestinal distress), and a recommendation for almsgiving. These remedies provide a set of widely efficacious substances, objects, and activities which work to enlist divine aid in the protection of the household and the woman herself, as well as to act directly on her psychophysical condition.

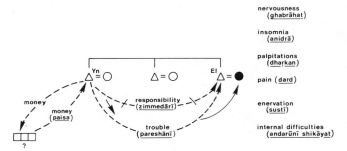

Fig. 4. The client's situation

These four cases indicate that an important part of astrological counseling involves the construction of images of the client's situation. The four situations presented here reflect a North Indian concept of the person as comprised of four aspects—body, mind, and family and community relationships. Both astrological classifications and the divinatory dialogues into which these classifications enter, reflect and appeal to a notion of a whole person of mutually articulated aspects, on the analogy of celestial conjunctions whose components take on meaning by virtue of their configurative relationships. The theory of the person as a system of four interrelated aspects makes the person conceptually continuous with the social world, thus deemphasizing the individual/society dichotomy which prevails in many areas of Western social and medical thought.

This holistic orientation is also formed by the continuity between person and situation which is emphasized in astrological hermeneutics. The situation in its multiform configurations locates the person in a focused set of relevances; while these relevances may change through time (both in the value of single relevances and in their configurative articulations), there is nonetheless a broader set of experiential categories—the variously articulated categories of mind, body, and family and community relationships—out of which are organized the configurative perceptions of new (and recurring) personal situations. These two features—an interrelationship among the aspects of the person and an articulation of person and situation—constitute a form of holism which shows close parallels with the holistic features which Lock (1980) identifies in East Asian medicine in Japan.

An important aspect of astrological counseling—one which is derived directly from its holistic formulation of person and situation—is its attention to the affective dimensions of human experience. Affect is dealt with not as a private internal phenomenon but rather as a socially sustained dimension of personal existence. This poses a striking contrast with Kleinman's (1980) findings from Taiwan, where there is an apparent lack of expression of the affective dimensions of personal problems in various psychotherapeutic settings. In the images of personal situations constructed in astrological counseling, affective experiences simultaneously modulate and are modulated by familial and social relationships. The person's natural involvement in family and community makes the affective and physical conditions of the members of his sociofamilial world important components in the organization of his own situation. In some situations, it may be the physical or affective condition of a kinsman or community member, as well as the physical or affective state of the person himself, which is construed as part of the dynamic structure of the situation.

The meaningfulness of astrological counseling is further enhanced by the style of language which is used in the practitioner-client dialogue. Counseling is conducted in a language which is replete with what Geertz (1976), following Kohut, has discussed as "experience-near" concepts. There do not seem to be the same sharp differences between therapy-style language and family-style or everyday-style language which Labov and Fanshel (1977) describe for Western psychotherapeutic conversations. Clients and astrologers talk informally in a language whose analytic constructs (such as destiny, person, situation, planetary influence, time cycles, and so on) do not represent abstract formulations alien to the language of everyday life. The holistic concept of person and the comprehensive projective schema embedded in astrological discourse work to facilitate an open-ended communication between practitioner and client.

Conclusion

The study of concepts of the person in the context of healing offers a perspective on the nature of order and meaning in therapeutic interactions. What is methodologically important in the present account is that four indigenously recognized aspects of the person—mind, body, and family and community relationships—are presented as components of a single conceptual system. And concepts of the situation are treated as symbolic entities of the same order as person-concepts. Together the concepts of person and situation appear to constitute key categories for the perception and treatment of a wide range of socioexistential problems, thus deeply informing the meaningfulness of experience in everyday life and the experience of meaningfulness in astrological counseling.

This approach cautions against the use of models of sickness as a framework for the analysis of counseling processes. While analytic perspectives oriented to the study of sickness may facilitate our understanding of universal disease processes and their culture-specific encodings in illness experience, they may at the same time have less utility in the cross-cultural study of counseling processes whose catchment of ailments and problems is considerably broader than sickness experiences in the strict sense. From a socioexistential perspective, divinatory counseling processes, such as astrological therapy, encompass a wide range of problems, of which disease is an important but non-diacritical component. Focusing descriptively and analytically on the symbolic construction of personal situations appears to provide a more complete way of conceptualizing the therapeutic goals and accomplishments of divinatory counseling.

South Asia's plural medical and counseling systems offer a rich field for the exploration of cultural perceptions of problematic life-experiences. The study of the cultural structures which inform these therapeutic traditions can guide us into the subtle underpinnings of everyday life and the subjectively construed dilemmas of disorder which mark the lives of ordinary North Indians. Descriptions of such key concepts as person and situation offer a set of generalizable analytic notions which may be useful in the study of other ethnomedical traditions. For instance, from the Indian context, the concept of the person as composed of four mutually coincident aspects may provide a broader frame of reference for the study of other medical and counseling systems than does the biomedical view. At a more general level, the exploration of concepts of person and situation in the context of astrological counseling serves to highlight broad themes in the Indian understanding of life-experience, especially a *socioexistential* orientation to personal order and disorder which helps to explain why, as Medard Boss reports (1965: 48), many Indian students of psychiatry feel a marked affinity for phenomenological approaches to the conceptualization of personal distress and its treatment.

NOTES

1   Concepts of the situation can also be explored in the context of Indian literature. For instance, the Hindi stories of Premchand provide excellent views of "situations" in Indian life. See Zide et al (1962) for a collection of these stories.

2   These ontological distinctions are embedded in social scientific perspectives which define culture as a set of beliefs and values and society as a system of social relations. Schneider (1976) provides a discussion of this problem
    These distinctions have been reproduced in various ways in the field of medical anthropology. For instance, in a recent overview of the field (see Lieban 1977), indigenous concepts of disease, body, and so on, in other words, "cultural" factors, come under the heading of "ethnomedicine," while social factors are dealt with under the headings of "epidemiology" and "medical aspects of social systems" (here primarily "sanctions" and "deviance").

3   These ontological distinctions are found, for instance, in Kleinman's recent work (1980:24-44; 133-145), most strikingly in his exposition of levels or types of reality.

4   Comaroff (1980) presents a different way of approaching problems of person, order, and therapy.

5   Studies of divination by Hsu (1976), Tseng (1976), Carstairs and Kapur (1976), Kleinman (1980), and Perinbanayagam (1981) use strongly psychological or psychiatric frameworks.

6   Turner's (1975) account of Ndembu divination provides an excellent picture of the experientially grounded meanings of the objects in the diviner's basket.

7   See Pugh (1982) for a fuller comparison of astrological therapy and Western psychotherapy and counseling, particularly "brief" or "time-limited" psychotherapy.

8   The 1971 Census of India gives a breakdown of the population of Banaras by religion, as follows: Hindu, 448,767; Muslim, 153,314; Christian, 2,006; Sikh, 1,712; Jain, 788; and Buddhist, 117.

9   Pugh (1981) provides a fuller account of astrology and divination among both Hindus and Muslims in Banaras.

10 This section is based on exegetical materials which I collected from Banaras astrologers and learned men, and on my observations of the advisory interactions between these practitioners and their clients. In their explanations of essential aspects of astrology, astrologers and diviners sometimes referred to charts and descriptive passages in almanacs and basic astrology texts. Some of the texts to which they referred are: *Jyotishdarpana* (Gupta n.d.), *Laghujātakam* (Varahamihira 1969), and *Intakhāb al-najūm* (1873). The charts in this section represent my own summations of these various discussions.

11 This template is conceptualized either as an internal template, that is, a code which the planetary realm imprints in the person's self at the time of birth, or as an external template, that is, a patterned trajectory of planetary influences in which the person is implicated by virtue of the time and place of his birth.

REFERENCES

Boss, Medard
  1965 *A Psychiatrist Discovers India*. London: Oswald Wolff.
Carstairs, G. M. and R. L. Kapur
  1976 *The Great Universe of Kota: Stress, Change, and Mental Disorder in an Indian Village*. Berkeley: University of California Press.
Census of India
  1971 Part II-C. Social and Cultural Tables. Uttar Pradesh. Pp. 62-63.
Chang, Yunshik
  1977 "The Urban Korean as Individual." *Korea Journal* 17(5): 49-57.
Comaroff, Jean
  1980 "Healing and the Cultural Order: the Case of the Barolong buu Ratshidi of Southern Africa." *American Ethnologist* 7(4): 637-657.
Dumont, Louis
  1970 *Homo Hierarchicus*. Chicago: University of Chicago Press.
Fortes, Meyer
  1976 "Foreward." *In* J. B. Loudon (ed.), *Social Anthropology and Medicine*. New York: Academic Press. Pp. ix-xx.
Geertz, Clifford
  1973 "Person, Time, and Conduct in Bali." *In* Clifford Geertz, *The Interpretation of Cultures*. New York: Basic Books. Pp. 360-411.
  1976 "'From the Native's Point of View': On the Nature of Anthropological Understanding." *In* Keith H. Basso and Henry A. Selby (eds.), *Meaning in Anthropology*. Albuquerque: University of New Mexico Press. Pp. 221-237.
Goffman, Erving
  1974 *Frame Analysis: An Essay on the Organization of Experience*. Cambridge: Harvard University Press.
Gupta, Vasudev
  n.d. *Jyotishdarpana* [The Mirror of Astrology]. Varanasi: Thakur Prasad and Sons.
Horton, Robin
  1967 "African Traditional Thought and Western Science." *Africa* 37(1-2): 50-71; 155-187.
Hsu, Jin
  1976 "Counseling in the Chinese Temple: A Psychological Study of Divination by Chien Drawing." *In* William Lebra (ed.), *Culture-Bound Syndromes, Ethnopsychiatry, and Alternate Therapies*. Honolulu: University Press of Hawaii. Pp. 210-221.
Inden, Ronald B. and Ralph W. Nicholas
  1977 *Kinship in Bengali Culture*. Chicago: University of Chicago Press.
Intakhāb al-najūm [Astrological Extracts]
  1873 Lucknow: Matba' Munshi Tej Kumar Press.

JANSEN, G.
    1973   *The Doctor-Patient Relationship in an African Tribal Society.* Assen, the Netherlands: Van
            Gorcum.
JANZEN, John M.
    1978   *The Quest for Therapy in Lower Zaire.* Berkeley: University of California Press.
KLEINMAN, Arthur M.
    1980   *Patients and Healers in the Context of Culture: An Exploration of the Borderland between An-
            thropology, Medicine, and Psychiatry.* Berkeley: University of California Press.
LABOV, William and David FANSHEL
    1977   *Therapeutic Discourse: Psychotherapy as Conversation.* New York: Academic Press.
LEWIS, Gilbert
    1975   *Knowledge of Illness in a Sepik Society.* London: Athlone Press.
    1976   "A View of Sickness in New Guinea." *In* J. B. Loudon (ed.), *Social Anthropology and
            Medicine.* New York: Academic Press. Pp. 49-103.
LIEBAN, Richard W.
    1977   "The Field of Medical Anthropology." *In* David Landy (ed.), *Culture, Disease, and
            Healing.* New York: Macmillan. Pp. 13-31.
LOCK, Margaret
    1980   *East Asian Medicine in Urban Japan.* Berkeley: University of California Press.
MARRIOTT, McKim
    1976   "Interpreting Indian Society: A Monistic Alternative to Dumont's Dualism." *Jour-
            nal of Asian Studies* 36(1): 189-195.
MARRIOTT, McKim and Robald B. INDEN
    1972   "An Ethnosociology of South Asian Caste Systems." Paper presented at the
            American Anthropological Association Meetings, Toronto, December 1972.
McHUGH, Peter
    1968   *Defining the Situation: The Organization of Meaning in Social Interaction.* New York: Bobbs-
            Merrill Company.
ORTNER, Sherry B.
    1978   *Sherpas Through Their Rituals.* Cambridge: Cambridge University Press.
PARSONS, Talcott
    1951   *The Social System.* New York: The Free Press.
PERINBANAYAGAM, R. S.
    1981   "Self, Other, and Astrology: Esoteric Therapy in Sri Lanka." *Psychiatry* 44: 69-79.
PUGH, Judy F.
    1981   Person and Experience: the Astrological System of North India. Unpublished Ph.D.
            dissertation, University of Chicago, Department of Anthropology.
    1983   "Astrological Counseling in Contemporary India." *Culture, Medicine and Psychiatry* 7:
            1-21.
ROSALDO, Michelle Z.
    1980   *Knowledge and Passion: Ilongot Notions of Self and Social Life.* Cambridge: Cambridge
            University Press.
SCHNEIDER, David M.
    1976   "Notes toward a Theory of Culture." *In* Keith H. Basso and Henry A Selby (eds.),
            Meaning in Anthropology. Albuquerque: University of New Mexico Press. Pp.
            197-220.
SCHUTZ, Alfred
    1967   *The Phenomenology of the Social World.* Evanston: Northwestern University Press.
TSENG, Wen-Shing
    1976   "Folk Psychotherapy in Taiwan." *In* William Lebra (ed.), *Culture-Bound Syndromes,
            Ethnopsychiatry, and Alternate Therapies.* Honolulu: University Press of Hawaii. Pp.
            164-178.
TURNER, Victor
    1975   *Revelation and Divination in Ndembu Ritual.* Ithaca: Cornell University Press.

VARAHAMIHIRA
1969 *Laghujātakam* [Abridged Nativity]. With Hindi commentary. Vasudev (ed.). Varanasi: Thakur Prasad and Sons.
ZIDE, Norman H. et al (eds.)
1962 *A Premchand Reader*. Honolulu: University of Hawaii East-West Center Press.

The Sufi as Saint, Curer, and Exorcist in Modern Pakistan*

KATHERINE EWING

University of Chicago, Chicago, U.S.A.

As PART OF FOLK ISLAM, Sufis and the Sufi Orders have come to play an important role in the healing process in all Muslim societies. The idiom of cure in most cases involves the ideas of possession, trance, and wondrous deeds; in other words, interpersonal intervention through the influence of spiritual forces. The forms which this healing takes and the definition and role of the Sufi in the healing process, however, vary from culture to culture within the Muslim world.

In this paper I will examine the nature of the relationship between the Sufi and the layman in Pakistani folk Islam in order to discover how curing is defined and effected within this symbolic and social context. I will discuss first how the social context of Sufi as "living saint" is created ritually and how this context defines in general terms the nature of the relationship between the curer and his patient. I will then go on to discuss the actual techniques of curing and how they link the religious system of meaning with the distress of the patient through symbolic articulation of the distress and its transformation into "cure" through the manipulation of symbols.

Crapanzano (1973), in his examination of the practices of the Hamadsha, a Sufi brotherhood in Morocco, as a system of psychotherapy, concludes that the primary agent of healing is not the curer. Rather, membership in the brotherhood as a group and participation in its group activity of ritual possession and trance are more crucial in the curing process. He stresses that the patient-curer relationship *per se* is not the source of efficacy of the cure:

> I am suggesting rather than neither a deep transference relationship with archaic features nor an important personal bond is established between patient and curer. Whatever transference is established is immediately deflected to supernatural agents — the saints and jnun. Even the power of the curer is conceived in supernatural terms, in terms of baraka (Crapanzano 1973: 217).

* *Acknowledgments*. This paper was originally presented at the 31st Annual Meeting of the Association for Asian Studies, held in Los Angeles, March 1979. It is based on fieldwork conducted in Lahore, Pakistan in 1975-77. My research was supported by a grant from the American Institute of Pakistan Studies and an award from the Committee on Southern Asian Studies at the University of Chicago. I would like to thank McKim Marriott, Ralph Nicholas, and Vincent Crapanzano for helpful criticisms and comments on earlier drafts of this paper.

Though many of the symbols used in the curing process, such as *baraka* (divine blessing) and *jinn* (spirit or demon; *jnun* is the Arabic plural) are identical among the Hamadsha of Moroco and the *Pirs* of Pakistan, the place of the Sufi both in the symbolic system and in the social context of the cure is radically different. According to Crapanzano's description, the organization of the Hamadsha emphasizes the brotherhood, i.e., relations among approximate equals. The leadership of the local order is an elected office. Among the Hamadsha, the saint is a distant, long-dead figure, and neither his descendants nor the leaders of the order have a status comparable to that of the saint.

Sufism in Pakistan, in contrast, focuses in both its popular and esoteric forms on the dyadic relationship between the *Pir*, who is regarded as a living saint, and each of his followers. Like the Moroccans, Pakistanis also assign great importance to the shrines of dead saints, but they make no fundamental distinction between these saints and those now living. The practice of Sufism has allowed certain men to become saints. The saint, by performing specific disciplines prescribed by the Sufi Order of which he is a member, has had *baraka* (God's blessing) bestowed upon him. The saint radiates this *baraka*, as does his grave after his death. Contact with this *baraka* is extremely beneficial to the ordinary man; it both facilitates his ultimate salvation and helps to ward off malevolent influences in this life. The saint is able to create an open channel between God and the world, and *baraka* is what flows through this channel. By coming into contact with a saint, whether living or dead, the follower himself comes closer to God.

The fundamental continuity between the shrines and the living saints in Pakistan is symbolized and enacted in several ways. The dress and general appearance of the *Pir*, for example, are explicity saintly and are believed to be a replication of the manner of dress of the Prophet Muhammad. The typical *Pir* is readily recognizable: he is middle-aged or older; he has silver or white hair and a neatly trimmed beard; he dresses completely in white and wears a white turban as well.

The importance of the details of appearance as a part of the embodiment of the concept of *Pir* (saint) is revealed in the dreams of followers and others, in which the narrator knows that he has dreamed of a saint because of the appearance of the stranger in his dream. In the dream, the saint is inevitably described as wearing white clothes and as having a beard, a fair complexion, and a kind smiling face. The *Pirs* whom I met did have faces that were markedly relaxed and gently smiling. There was, in fact, a characteristic facial expression which these *Pirs* tended to assume or lapse into when in mediation or listening to the problems of their followers. Their gaze was direct and almost unblinking, or, alternatively, the eyes were almost closed. In a society in which women are veiled and honourable men avoid looking at them, this gaze is unusual and affirms the extraordinary status of the *Pir*, who is different from ordinary men.

Many Pakistanis stress the importance of the saint's being a Sayyid, a descendant of the Prophet, but even more important than this blood tie to the

Prophet, is the direct spiritual descent of the living *Pir* from Sufi *Pirs* before him. It is this descent that links him with a specific Sufi Order and legitimates his position as a saint. The visitor is immediately assured of this spiritual descent when he enters the *baithak* (reception room) of the typical *Pir*. Hanging on the wall, amid pictures of the *ka'abah* in Mecca and tombs of other saints, there will be a framed copy of the *shajra* of the *Pir*. This is a chart which traces his spiritual descent in the Sufi to which he belongs. The *Pir* might also have installed a glass case in which the turban and other possessions of the Pir who initiated him into the Order are displayed.

The *baithak* itself is important for creating the context in which a saint receives his followers and for emphasizing the continuity between the living saint and the saints who are honoured at shrines. Most people see him in a room specially furnished for this purpose. This room is normally devoid of furniture except reed mats on the floor, a small carpet on which the *Pir* sits, and bolsters for him to lean against. Often, there is also a trunk in which books and papers are kept, and a *Pir* who is also a *hakim* (a practitioner of indigenous medicine) will have the appropriate medicines and other equipment beside him. When visitors enter, they leave their shoes outside the door. When they leave, they back out of the door, facing the *Pir* in the same manner that they would exit from a shrine. The saint always sits in the same spot, and in the case of the saint who receives his followers out of doors, he will if possible, be buried in precisely the same spot where he passed his days. The *baithak* thus becomes transformed into a shrine.

It is in this highly ritualized environment, embodying traditions that extend back to the Prophet, that the visitor/patient first encounters the *Pir*. All of the characteristics of the *Pir*, his appearance, facial expression, spiritual genealogy, and the setting in which his followers interact with him, combine to create a specific set of expectations in the visitor. This set of expectations and beliefs must be kept in mind when analyzing the nature of the relationship between the *Pir* and his followers.

Overtly, there does not appear to be anything approaching the intimacy of the Western psychotherapeutic process in this interaction. Because of the brevity of the contact, which I will describe below, one might be temped to conclude, as Crapanzano does in the very different case of the Hamadsha of Morocco, that there is no deep transference relationship. Among the Hamadsha, the transference is deflected away from the curer onto spiritual agents such as dead saints and *jnun*. In Pakistan, in contrast, the *Pir* is himself an agent, who, even though still embodied, can act spiritually (*ruhani tor pur*) in the world. The visitor who comes seeking advice or a cure believes that the *Pir* is a direct channel of communication with god and that the *Pir's* presence and awareness are not limited in the way that the senses of ordinary people are. For example, I was speaking to a follower of one *Pir* who was seated in the next room. Though we were well out of earshot of the *Pir*, the follower was circumspect in his answers because, as he said, the *Pir* was able to hear anything that went on. He could even sense everything we were thinking. When the visitor comes before the *Pir*, he expects the *Pir* to be able to discover at a glance precisely what the trouble is. The *Pir* can read instantly the state of one's body and soul. Because of this power of the *Pir*, it is not considered necessary for the *Pir* to engage in a long interaction with his follower.

The visitor gives a brief account of the specific problem that is troubling him. These accounts usually are as formulaic as the *Pir's* responses are. In the course of my observation of one *Pir*, I heard many people narrate their complaints. These complaints included such things as sickness, infertility, problems with one's job, and fear of failure on an exam. As a few perceptive followers pointed out, however, the specific complaint which the visitor recounts is often not the "real" trouble. The actual problem may be a vague anxiety, or it may be something that the person is too embarrassed to talk about. Therefore, he or she presents a standard problem instead.

Such misrepresentation is especially common when, as is often the case, a spouse or other relative has accompanied the troubled person. Usually they will come forward together to sit before the *Pir*. In one instance which I witnessed, two sisters-in-law visited a *Pir*. One complained of fatigue and the other asked for an amulet for her child. In this particular case, it was a quiet day, and one of the women was able to linger behind until she was alone with the *Pir* (and me). She then revealed that her sister-in-law was sleeping with her husband. The *Pir* gave her advice on how to be more appealing to her husband. Candidness in this situation was, at least in my observation, unusual. A visitor is rarely alone with the *Pir*.

The standardization of complaints may also be a product of the vocabulary of distress and of underlying assumptions about the causes of distress. This distress may be, in our way of looking at it, either "physical" or "mental"—the two cannot be separated phenomenologically. In Pakistani thought, health is interpersonal. Happiness prevails when people, especially relatives, behave properly towards one another. Proper behavior is defined in terms of being a good Muslim, and includes expectations such as the obedience and respect of juniors toward elders and the proper channeling of love throughout the family. When these expectations are violated, there is unhappiness, and unhappiness leads to illness or even death. All such problems are ultimately a violation of spiritual order. The patient merely names the part of the body or area of his life where he perceives his distress to be concentrated. Because of the belief in the omniscience of the *Pir*, the follower does not consider it to be necessary to represent his or her problem in detail. The *Pir* will penetrate to the heart of the problem regardless of what is said. Thus, in the case mentioned above, the woman, even if she had not seen the *Pir* alone, would have probably assumed that he had been able to discern the difficulty anyway and that he would have taken her underlying difficulty into account when writing an amulet for her.

There may be forty or more followers seated at the feet of the *Pir* at any one time. One by one, the followers (the majority being women) approach the *Pir*, sit before him, and quickly state their problems. The *Pir* writes an amulet (*ta'wiz*), blows on it and on the patient, and mutters a verse of the Qur'an while handing the amulet to the patient. He tells the patient to pray in a specified way and gives instructions for use of the amulet. Specific techniques vary from *Pir* to *Pir*, but whichever technique the *Pir* uses, it is standardized, so that he treats each patient in basically the same way.

The simplest and most frequent technique used by the *Pir* is *dam* (literally, "breath"). In this technique, the saint simply utters a verse of the Qur'an, quickly and inaudibly, and then blows on the patient. If a specific part of the body is the source of trouble, he will focus his breath on that area. Otherwise, he will blow on the patient's bowed head or sweep from the top of the head down to the floor. In this act the *baraka* of God, channeled through the saint, is transferred to the patient in the breath. By uttering a specific verse of the Qur'an first, the powers of this verse are also transferred.

A slightly more elaborate version of this technique is known as *dam-pani* (literally, "breath-water"). Here, the *Pir* utters a Qur'anic verse and blows on a vial of water instead of blowing directly on the patient. He then gives precise instructions on when and how this water is to be used. Usually, the water is to be drunk three times a day after prayers for a specified number of days. In this technique the blessing is transferred to the water and can thus be taken home in order for it to be administered to a third party, such as a sick child. One *Pir*, in his own variant of this technique, sits with a tray of rock salt and a hammer before him. While the patient is telling him what the difficulty is, he is gently tapping at a chunk of salt. He offers some advice, blows on the patient, then quickly licks the salt, wraps it in a small piece of newspaper, and hands it to the patient.

Another standard technique, mentioned above, is the writing of an amulet. The logic of the effectiveness of an amulet is essentially the same as that of *dam* and *dam-pani*, but the art of writing an amulet is tied in with an elaborate traditional "luminous knowledge" (*nuri 'ilm*). In this system, each letter of the alphabet is assigned a number, based upon the positions of the letter in the alphabet. In the writing of an amulet, the *Pir* chooses a particular verse of the Qur'an or name of God, the choice of which is determined by the nature of the complaint of the patient. He assigns the initial letter of the name of God a number and uses this number as the foundations of a magic square. Many *Pirs* personalize the amulet by asking the name of the patient and of the patient's mother. They then use the first letter of each of these names in the writing of the amulet. Other techniques may also be used for the writing of an amulet, but in every case, what is stressed is the complexity of the system on which amulet writing is based. Because of this complexity, the expertise of the *Pir* is essential.

The expertise and authority which are revealed by the ability to write amulets are even more crucial in the case of the exorcism ritual, which the *Pir* is occasionally called upon to perform. Often, a person comes or is brought to a *Pir* with the complaint that she (it is usually a woman) is possessed by a *jinn* or some other spirit. As Crapanzano and others have suggested, possession by a spirit is a way of representing in symbolic terms deep and inchoate emotional troubles of the patient. South Asian Muslim exorcism rites clearly illustrate how such a symbolic transformation takes place.

As a result of his closeness to God, the saint also has direct access to the power of God. It is this spiritual power which enables him to control other supernatural beings such as *jinn* and thus to perform exorcisms. In the performance of an exorcism, both Punjabi, the local language, and Arabic, the language of the Qur'an, are used. The organizational frame of the ritual is created by the commands, questions, and responses in Punjabi of the curer and patient. By his utterances, the *Pir* is creating order in the ritual and tying in the conceptual scheme of *nuri 'ilm* with specific ritual actions. These utterances have an immediate communicative function: they inform both the patient and observers of the significance of ongoing ritual actions and Arabic utterances. Thus the following quotation taken from a description of a nineteenth century exorcism consists of a command issued to the demon intended to make the demon manifest itself, which follows an Arabic spell intended to produce the same effect:

> Having read the Arabic incantation, the exorcist is to add, "Whatever it be that has taken possession of the body of such a one, come out of him, come out of him" (Shurreef 1973: 219).

This command may be explained, not only as aiding in producing the result of making the demon appear, but as communicating to the audience and patient that this is the intended effect of the previous spell. It is the Arabic spell which is intended to produce the magical effect. The imperative in Punjabi, by directly addressing specific demons, serves to focus the power inherent in the Arabic spell onto those specific demons and to specify the exorcist's desires. The Arabic draws upon God's power in a generalized manner, whereas the imperative in Punjabi specifies what the exorcist wants to do with that power. Their reference is to God, His actions and attributes, basically assertations of His character and power. Most are not directly supplications addressed to God requesting His aid. Their ritual efficacy may be said to derive from the fact not that they are words addressed to God, enlisting His aid, but rather they are words of God, as revealed to the Prophet Muhammed. They create their effects, not by conveying a meaning to which listeners are to directly respond, but by the power inherent in the words themselves as God's words. Their meaning is often only marginally related to the event at hand.

Tambiah, in analyzing the structure and function of exorcism, says:

> Here the exorcist as protagonist must appear more terrible and powerful than the demon inside the patient, and the secretly muttered spells not only constitute the language the demons can understand, but more importantly, contributed to the image of the exorcist's own power (Tambiah 1968: 179).

In the case of Muslim exorcism, the control of "God's words" by the exorcist gives him such a power over the demons. Tambiah speaks of "transference" of the power of a spell to the final recipient through the ritual use of objects (Tambiah 1968: 190), a concept which he later refined and label "persuasive analogy" (1973).

> The objects are chosen on the basis of similarity and difference to convey meaning. From the performative perspective, the action consists of an operation done on an object-symbol to make an imperative and realistic transfer of its properties to the recipient (Tambiah 1973: 222).

In the case of the Punjabi Muslim exorcism ritual, there appear to be a series of actions which transfer the properties of a ritual object to the patient. In this ritual, however, it is often merely the Arabic utterances, i.e., Qur'anic verses and the Attributes of God, which are the focus of activity. The central ritual "object-symbols" are thus not material objects with specific physical properties. Instead, the Arabic words themselves are being treated as concrete objects whose properties can be transferred to the patient by mechanical means. The intention of the ritual is to cause the power of these Arabic words to operate within the patient, regardless of whether he actually hears them or not.

There are several media of transfer. These media of transfer are precisely the devices which are used in the everyday ritual activity of the *Pir*, namely, breath, water, and written verses of the Qur'an.

A common practice, once it is ascertained that the demon is actually in possession of the patient, is to prevent him from escaping by tying a knot in the patient's hair. The *Pir* then recites a verse from the Qur'an and blows on the knot. In this case it would seem that the knot is literally intended to hold in the demon, which would otherwise escape through the head of the patient. Purely mechanical actions, however, will not restrain a demon, whose essential nature is spiritual. The spell allows the *Pir's* mechanical actions to be dominant over the demon. Similarly, the *Pir* will read a spell over a stick before beating the possessed patient, in order to make the demon answer his questions. Observers claim that the severe beating causes no physical injury to the patient. The logic appears to be that the associations of a spell with a physical action and a material object transforms the actions so that it is effective in a spiritual, non-corporeal realm.

In the Pakistani cosmological system, the *jinn* and humans have parallel genealogies and worlds and are distinguished essentially by the opposition corporeal/non-corporeal. They can operate independently of each other without interference, but from time to time the *jinn* attempt to cross the boundary. The spells are the mediators which enable man to cross the boundary between the physical and the spiritual and thus to meet the *jinn* and take action in relation to them. A *jinn*, incorporated temporarily in the patient, is at the intersection of the two domains, occupying both, and the exorcist's actions, to be effective, must also be both corporeal and spiritual.

Shurreef's description of the successful conclusion of an exorcism is a particularly vivid illustration of this conjunction of the spiritual and the physical. At the moment the demon decides to leave the body of the patient, he runs away from the exorcist, but the exorcist maintains a grasp on the patient's hair, thus blocking the demon's route of escape. The exorcist plucks out one or two of the hairs, "and reading some established spell over them, puts them into a bottle and corks it up; whereupon the patient's devil is supposed to be imprisoned therein" (Shurreef 1973: 222). The exorcist, with the help of the spells, which make his actions effective on a non-corporeal being, thus imprisons the *jinn* in a material form, the hairs. Trapped in a material form, he is trapped in a physical space.

In terms of the patient's perception of the ritual and its effectiveness, his disturbance or illness has been explained and conquered by the exorcist and then externalized. The patient can see his illness, previously formless and powerful within him, now outside of himself, trapped in a bottle. The *Pir* performing physical actions has been effective in a spiritual realm, thus acting as a mediator between the two. The *Pir* has a physical body, yet he can operate in a spiritual realm, like the *jinn*. Before the exorcism, the *jinn*, or illness, was not embodied and thus was impossible for the patient to control. The goal of the ritual is to give the illness (represented as a *jinn*) physical substance, permanent incorporation outside the patient. Throughout the ritual the *Pir* incorporates the incorporeal in the form of words. He treats them as objects and causes them to make physical contact with the patient and the demon. His ritual action thus symbolizes the desired final effect: the spiritual illness becomes physical hair trapped in a bottle.

From the perspective of a participant in a Muslim exorcism, the force of the Arabic spell is not seen merely as speech, effective by conveying meaning. It is instead mechanically effective on a spiritual agent in a manner analogous to the way a non-symbolic physical action is effective upon a physical being. This analogy is really the "persuasive analogy" of the ritual. The participants in the ritual are to be persuaded that these formalized utterances are not merely words, but are "just like" physical actions and thus will have the effectiveness that physical actions do.

The elaborate system of "luminous knowledge" (*nuri 'ilm*) of exorcism is a set of categories designed to strengthen the analogy created in the exorcism by presenting a relatively consistent cognitive scheme to which the ritual actions can be referred. Levi-Strauss, in analyzing a shamanistic cure, explains in a similar manner the source of effectiveness of such a cure (Levi-Strauss 1967). The procedure of asking the possessed patient specific information about the *jinn*, such as the *jinn's* name, astrological sign, etc., serves to explicitly tie in the patient's specific illness with the general cosmological scheme, to force the patient to conceptualize it in those terms, and to remind all present of the cognitive scheme and its effectiveness. The exorcism ritual itself consists of an elaborate system of mediations of the boundary between spiritual and physical, with utterances accomplishing the conceptual transformation of an uncontrollable spiritual illness into a controlled and knowable physical object, reflecting the principle that what is known and named is under man's control.

Explication of the exorcism ritual makes the process of symbolic transformation explicit because of its extreme conjunction of the physical and the spiritual, the cognitive and the emotional. But the *Pir* performs the same symbolic operations every day when he blows a Qur'anic verse onto a patient or writes an amulet. With respect to even the most mundane disease, its cause and its cure, the physical and the mental or spiritual are not differentiated. Possession by a spirit need not take the form of madness; it may be a wasting disease or a chill or some other chronic ailment. Just as a "physical" disease such as this may be assigned a spiritual cause, a case of spiritual distress or anxiety may be described as a physical symptom, such as a pain in the stomach. The *Pir* operates in both the physical and spiritual domains. He may even have a supply of traditional medicines which he dispenses along with the amulets. But in every treatment, the position of the *Pir* as spiritual agent is essential to the process of cure, because only he can perceive and channel the power and blessing of God, moving it from the realm of the spiritual to the physical world.

The role of the Sufi Saint as spiritual agent and the relationship between Sufi and follower as reflected in the curing process is linked to the whole organization of the Sufi orders in Pakistan, which stresses an intense dyadic relationship between saint and follower. This organization provides a therapeutic structure which is congenial with the culturally patterned expectations of the Pakistani patient in distress.

REFERENCES

CRAPANZANO, Vincent
    1973   *The Hamadsha: A Study in Moroccan Ethnopsychiatry*. Berkeley: University of California Press.
LEVI-STRAUSS, Claude
    1967   "The Effectiveness of Symbols." *In* Claude Levi-Strauss, *Structural Anthropology*. Garden City, New York: Doubleday (Anchor Books).
SHURREEF, Jaffur
    1973   *Qanoon-e-Islam, or The Customs of the Mussalmans of India*. G. A. Herklots, trans. Lahore: Al-Irshad Reprints. (orig. pub. London 1832).
TAMBIAH, Stanley
    1968   "The Magical Power of Words." *Man* 3: 175-208.
    1973   "Form and Meaning of Magical Acts: A Point of View." *In* Robin Horton and Ruth Finnegan (eds.), *Modes of Thought*. London: Faber and Faber.

The Pulse as an Icon in Siddha Medicine

E. VALENTINE DANIEL

University of Washington, Seattle, U.S.A.

THE SIDDHA MEDICAL SYSTEM, along with Ayurveda and Yunani, constitute the three formalized traditional medical systems of India. Practitioners of Siddha medicine claim that their system is not derived from Ayurveda but from the writings of the eighteen *cittars* who lived between the 10th and 15th centuries and composed cryptic verses in Tamil by means of which medical lore was preserved and transmitted down the ages (K. Zvelebil 1973: pp 218-236 and 1974: 54-57).

In Siddha medicine, as in Ayurveda, Yunani, and traditional Chinese medicines, the pulse is the sign *par excellence* for the diagnostician. Other signs, symptoms, and syndromes are ancillary to or corroborative of the significance of the pulse. In this essay,[1] following a brief description of the pulse-reading-technique of the siddha physician and an adumbration of the theory underlying it, I shall argue that a semeiotic approach to the pulse (*nāṭi*) betrays a fundamental difference between the systems of thought in Siddha medicine and biomedicine.

In Siddha medicine, the basis of all pathology is to be located in an imbalance of the three humors, bile (*pittam*), wind (*vāyu*), and phlegm (*kapam*). Conversely, an equilibrated state of these humors in a human being indicates a state of good health. The particular nature of the imbalance in a patient's body is determined by the reading of his or her pulse. The Siddha physician is trained to distinguish six different pulses rather than the single, diastolic-systolic pulse that the biomedical health-practitioner is known to identify. Of the six pulses, three are read from the right wrist and three from the left.

The Siddha physician takes a hold of the patient's right wrist in his left hand and places his index finger nearest the base of the thumb, on the inner side of the wrist, between the styloid process of the radius and the trapezium; his middle finger is placed next to the index finger, and the ring finger next to the middle finger. Each one of the three fingers senses or reads a different pulse. The index finger senses the pulse that indexes the wind humor, the middle finger, bile, and the ring finger, phlegm. These three pulses are held to pulsate at three distinguishably different rates. These rates are compared to the trotting of a chicken (wind), the leaping of a frog (bile), and the crawling of a snake (phlegm). The time-intervals between pulsations is called *naṭai* (pace or walk).

The *naṭai* of a pulse is employed to identify the distinctiveness of the three humoral pulses. Once this has been done, the physician attempts to sense in his fingertips the differential pressures exerted by these three pulses. These distinguishable pressures are called *eṭai* (weights). By comparing the *eṭai* of the three humor-indicating pulses in a person's wrist, the physician is able to determine which humor predominates in a person's system and which is or are inadequate or recessive.

The two quatrains[2] extant in the Siddha medical lore which describe the *eṭai* and *naṭai* as they are determined in the humoral pulsations are the following:

illayē vātam eṟilnaṭai kōṟiyām
ellaiyē pittam eṟumpum tavaḷai pōl
ollaiyē aiyam ūrntiṭum pāmpupōl
allaiyē kaṇṭinkarintavar cittarē
(Absent are the afflictions of wind when the chicken walks lightly,
The bounds of bile are known by the leaping of the frog,
And the crawling snake shys all quickness.
He who descerns this is a true Siddhar.)

varankiya vātam māttirai ontrākil
tarankiya pittam tannil araivāci
aranku kapantān aṭankiyē kālōṭil
viṟankiya cīvatrkup pisakontrum illaiyē
(If wind is measured as one unit in its prominence
And the amplitude of bile be half of that,
With sluggish phlegm a crawling fourth,
Then in whom these inhere is free of all care.)

To complicate matters further, the same operations of reading the *naṭai* and *eṭai* of the three humoral pulses are carried out on the other wrist of the patient as well, thereby giving the physician a total of six readings. Thus for each humor, there is a left aspect and a right aspect, yielding a total of six sub-humors. Each of the six sub-humors governs or compels (*iyakkutal*) a corresponding body tissue or body fluid (*tātu*) as shown below.

nāṭi (pulse)	*tātu* (body tissue)
Right wind	Blood
Right bile	Bone
Right phlegm	Flesh
Left wind	Fat/Marrow
Left bile	Nerve tissue/Skin
Left phlegm	Saliva

The only *tātu* (the seventh) that the pulse does not directly index is semen. In fact, semen being the carrier of the seed, and the seed the repository of all *tātus*, all six pulses collectively indicate the disposition of the seed or semen (See Daniel, 1984).

Apart from these six readings made available to the physician by the pulse of the patient, there are three stages or phases to each act of pulse-reading. The first is called the *stūla nilai* (the grossly sensory stage). *Stūla* is a concept that is usually associated with the body, as in *stūla śarīram* (the gross body), which refers to the outermost body sheath in the theory of the five body sheaths (*pañcamayakośa*). *Stūla* stands in complementary opposition to *sukṣma* or subtleness (from *sukṣma śarīram* or subtle body, the next outermost layer in the five body sheaths). Thus, *stūla* connotes something solid and tangible, in short, something objective. It is *objective* in the sense that it is *ob*servable (in this case by means of the sense of touch), and becomes as such because it presents itself as an *ob*stacle to the smooth, unobjected flow of the senses in pure potentia. At this stage of the reading of the pulse, the apparently "passive" fingertips of the physician, *ob*jects and *ob*jectifies the dynamic and hitherto unresisted flow of blood in the radial artery.

The second stage in the reading of the pulse is called *ul nilai* (the inner stage). In this stage or phase in the act of reading the pulse of a patient, the digital extremities of the physician that are in contact with the wrist of the patient are no longer "passive" or "inert" resisters as in the first stage, but rather, come alive with their own pulsations. In other words, the physician becomes aware of the rhythmic undulations of his own pulses in addition to the ones felt in the patient's radial artery. This stage is only an intermediary one in which the distinctly different pulsations of the patient and the physician are set out in palpable relief by means of the contrapuntal juxtaposition they are united in.

In the third stage, the physician modulates the *eṭai* and *naṭai* of his own pulses so that they become confluent and concordant with the pulses of the patient. This stage is called *cama nilai*, the state of equipoise. It is only at this stage that the Siddha physician believes that he "knows" the humoral disorder of the patient. The ability to bring his pulse into confluence with that of his patient is a skill which takes years to cultivate and is made possible only through years of apprenticeship under a preceptor. It is only after the physician has in this manner, experienced this phase or stage of "shared" pulsations that he is ready to release the wrist of his patient and begin drawing from his knowledge of text and verse for a prescription and advice.

Before we examine the semeiotic dimension of the Siddha art of pulse-reading I think it would be helpful if we briefly spelt out some of the major features of the semeiotic sign which will have a direct bearing on our analysis. To this task I now turn.

Structure of the Sign

Charles Sanders Peirce, the founder of modern semeiotics, conceived the sign as being constituted of three irreducible correlates: the representamen, the object and the interpretant. None of these correlates by itself constitutes the *meaning* of the sign but may be prescinded from each other and understood in terms of the different functional modes in which they enter into the triadic, meaningful, sign-relation.

> "A sign, or representamen, is a First which stands in such a genuine triadic relation to a Second, called its object, as to be capable of determining a Third, called its interpretant, to assume the same triadic relation to its object in which it stands itself to the same Object." (Peirce 1934: 2.274)[3]

A representamen in and of itself is not a full fledged sign but is only a sign in potentia. It becomes a completed sign when it chooses to represent something other than itself to something or somebody in some respect or capacity. That for which the representamen stands is the object. The object need not be a material thing. Rather, as its Latin root indicates, it is that which is thrown before the mind. "The Interpretant is another sign to which the represented object is addressed and by which its representation is interpreted. More generally it is the locus of interpretation and that by which a sign is linked to its context" (Deacon 1978: p. 147).

This linking of correlates entails a "leaping" or "jumping" activity between the correlates. Uexkull (1979) calls it a *Bedeutungssprung* which Eugene Baer (1982) translates as "a jump of meaning". Uexkull illustrates the *Bedeutungssprung* by employing the example of the telephone wherein there exists a non-causal relationship between electro-magnetic oscillations, the sounds, and the words and sentences uttered and heard. Baer notes the obvious similarity between Uexkull's semeiotic model and de Saussure's famous diagram illustrating the typical speech situation in which two interlocutors are involved. In the Saussurian scheme, non-causal but stable relations of meaning which presuppose a code that determines the system of meaning, entails physical, psychological, and physiological systems of signs at the same time. "Saussure's model ... presents meaning as a series of translations which, by way of coding, 'jump' from one universe of discourse to another" (p. 170). What is true for different systems of signs or even different universes of discourse is also true of the internal structure of the sign wherein three correlates are linked by a *Bedeutungssprung*. This much is obvious in so far that a system of signs or a universe of discourse is in its own right a sign writ large.

One of Peirce's greatest contributions to semeiotics is to be found in his two classifications of signs; the first, a system of nine signs and the second one of sixty six signs (See Peirce 2: 235-241; 1977: 160-166; Fitzgerald 1966; Weiss and Burks 1945). The value of these classifications is not to be found in the genius of his logic as an end in itself but in the fact that it provides us with a means of appreciating the multiple modes in which signs and correlates of signs are linked together, and furthermore, that it helps us understand the principles of the forces that motivate these links or *Bedeutungssprungs*.

In this essay I shall make but partial use of Peirce's first taxonomic classificaton of sign types to understand the semeiosis of pulsetaking. In this classification Peirce postulates three principles that motivate or impel the bringing together of a representamen and its object. These principles may be called iconicity, indexicality, and symbolization. The terms icon, index, and symbol, respectively, stand for the objects thus motivated.

In iconicity, object and representamen have some quality in common; some characteristic quality of the object being literally re-presented in the representamen. This sharing may range from partial resemblance, as in a diagram or image to a total identity with the object as in the case of an animal re-presenting the color and texture of its natural environment in its body in the well-known phenomenon of protective coloration.

In indexicality, there is no intrinsic sharing of qualities but instead, the object and representamen achieve their significant link by means of coincidence, contiguity, or cooccurrence. Indexes may range from instances in which the representamen embodies its own object directly, as in the case of a litmus paper turning red when dipped in an acidic solution, to conventionally determined contiguities such as the use of certain pronominal indexes in some languages to indicate high or low status of the addressee. Such status indexes along with a whole panoply of verbal indexes has been magnificently analyzed by Silverstein (1976).

In symbolization, convention (bereft of any significant resemblance of connection between object and representamen) is the principle that provides the motivating force for the *Bedeutungssprung*. And the defining feature of convention is its arbitrariness. The greater part of human languages is of the nature of symbols.

The sign and the pulse

In the context of the reading of the pulse in Siddha medicine, all three motivating principles are implicated. The conventional corpus of Siddha medicine as a tradition, as a body of knowledge, constitutes one system of signs, or universe of discourse; a system in which the dominant mode of signification is symbolic. The patient's pulse is another, a largely indexical system. So is the pulse of the physician. The movement of humors constitute yet another system. The translation of one system of signs into another, which is essentially what diagnosis (*gnosis* = knowledge, to know; *dia* = between, across), is all about, entails a *Bedeutungssprung*.

The three correlates that constitute the sign, "the patient,"[4] are: an imbalance of humors (as representamen), suffering (as object), and an abnormal pulse (as interpretant). Likewise, the sign, "the physician", is constituted of balanced humors (as representamen), an absence of suffering (as object) and a normal pulse (as interpretant).[5] The latter in itself may be divided into two parts or stages: the first, the "grossly sensory stage" when his own pulse is apparently inert, and the second, the "inner stage" when the pulse in his fingertips becomes active. In both instances, the "physician" as a sign, remains outside of and opposed to the "patient-sign." It is this very opposition that precipitate these two as *existent facts*, the one establishing the presence of the other and making this presence felt. Their contiguity makes them into indexical signs. The two interpretants (the pulses) by their very contact index each other, one as normal (first latently and then manifestly) and the other as abnormal. In so doing, however, they also reflexively index themselves internally; the abnormal pulse construing a meaningful link between imbalanced humors and suffering, and the normal pulse imposing a link between a balanced humoral state and non-suffering.

During what I have called the "gross sensory state," when the patient's pulse actively throbs against the passive fingertips of the physician, the indexical relationship that binds the two together may be thought of as being marked by a greater "distance" than during the "inner stage" when both physician's and patient's pulses pulsate contrapuntally. In the first stage the interdigitation is one between active effector and passive receptor. In the second stage indexical distance between the two signs is shortened. Even though the dominant signifying function remains indexical, a distinctly iconic component is seen to enter the sign relationship; both signs *share* the element of pulsation. Interdigitation turns into inosculation or anastomosis, so to speak. The clearly indexical sign is transformed into an indexical icon.

This leads into the next stage in which the two pulses do not pulsate contrapuntually but concurrently or confluently. The two signs become one; they become perfect icons of each other. At this moment of perfect iconicity, the physician may be said to have experienced in some sense the suffering as well as the humoral imbalance of the patient. It is the knowledge derived from this experience that makes him fit to return to his own symbolic tradition, the Siddha body of knowledge, to find therein the appropriate remedy to prescibe. In letting go of the wrist of the patient the physician's pulse is restored to its previous state. However, a trace of the experience remains in and informs his actions that follow.

The point I wish to stress here is that the epistemological if not empirical basis of pulse-reading in Siddha medicine provides for the possibility of neutralizing the great divide that separates physician from patient, even if only for a moment, at which time objectivity is replaced by consubjectivity.

The sign in biomedicine

In the biomedical universe of discourse, as is well known, "sign" is used, in the main, to contrast itself from "symptom," This use of the word "sign" in a marked sense is different from the sense in which it is used in Peircean semeiotics, a point which deserves to be noted in passing but one which will not play a crucial role in our present discussion. Symptoms are the expressed products of the patient's subjective experience, what he feels and at times what he thinks. The biomedical sign, on the other hand, is the objective indicator available to the physician's privilleged "gaze" (to borrow a concept from Foucault). And as Foucault has pointed out, at least since the eighteenth century, symptoms are worthy of attention only if they can either be reduced to and identified with disease, the *natural* object, or if they can be subsumed into the sign (1973: 93). The biomedical sign is the only sign worthy of being considered to be a biomedical sign. The zeal with which the medical profession carries this opinion masks the fact that the interpretative authority (the interpretant) which decides that a certain sign is an index in a universe of discourse (biomedical discourse) is itself largely conventional and symbolic. Biomedical texts are revered as compilations of indexical signs which are intended to eliminate "uncertainty." Scholars such as Renée Fox (1980) and David Sudnow (1967) who are humble enough to accept the inevitability of medical uncertainty and devote their efforts to coping with it as much as to reducing or transforming it are the exception rather than the rule. Even as brilliant a student of symbology as Susan Sontag, in her rich little book on *Illness as Metaphor* (1977), commits herself to the positivist task of ridding illness of all metaphor and thereby "liberating" it from all symbolic uncertainty. Her aim is to link illness or disease to its invariable and coincident indexical sign; no more, no less.

My criticism of biomedicine's unawareness of its symbolic (cultural and conventional) sources is no less applicable to traditional professional medical systems of India and elsewhere. One may even argue that scientific medicine's commitment to the empirical method and Popperian principles of falsification make "uncertainty" an integral part of its program. Paradoxically, however, it is in this very posture of scientistic smugness lies the danger of not being able to admit to the existence of uncertainties outside one's model, paradigm or episteme. Foucault's monumental studies on insanity (1965), the clinic (1973), and the penal system (1977), speak to this point.

There are other implications that derive from the centrality and sole governance of biomedical discourse by indexicality. In Peirce's scheme, the index, more than the icon or the symbol, foregrounds the *object* and the facticity of the object. Along with biomedicine's commitment to increase the quantity and power of indexical signs in one's discourse goes its corollary, *object*ification. The quest to positively identify a disease as "disease," as a thing, distinguished from the more subjective "illness" (see Hahn, this volume), is an instance of indexing and objectifying. The act of objectification itself has been appropriated by the sense of sight. If the history of medicine in the west shows us anything, it is this process of objectification through sight. The narrative technique, so much a part of the pre -and early 17th century country doctor, became increasingly subjugated to "observation," the observation of *things*, such as the outward appearance of the patient, his facial expression, his posture, skin color, manner of breathing, urine, stools, and blood. Sydenham's writings and journals cover the period of transition from a predominantly narration-dependent medicine to an observation dependent one. Even though Sydenham combined disease history and observation, he loathed to go so far as to entertain autopsy. Before observation, that is, before the "gaze," began to penetrate the body as a matter of course, Auenbrugger's digital percussion and Laennec's stethoscope had to prepare the way, and eventually, mediated ausculation established itself as a more successful auditory penetrant than percussion. In the move from narration to ausculation, verbal symbols were being replaced by non-verbal indexes. Ausculation, in fact, heralds in the objective physician in quite a dramatic way. No longer was it necessary for the physician to get snarled in and by the patient's experiences and symptoms but instead was able to isolate himself from the patient's "noises" and listen to the sounds produced in the patient, sounds to which the patient has no access and over which he has little control.

With the invention of the ophthalmoscope and the laryngoscope, the penetration of the "gaze" into the object (the patient) had become so commonplace that very few physicians doubted the aphorism, "To see is to believe." Photography made the replication of a patient's lesions in hundreds of glossy medical textbooks a reality, further alienating the patient from his own body. The microscope followed and the x-ray brought the century to a close, yielding to the "gaze" and its quest for indexical signs of disease a licence that knew no limits.

To repeat, Siddha, as well as other traditional Indian medical systems, are no more given to reflecting upon their *symbolic* roots than is biomedicine. I do hope that this will change. The current climate of ideological colonialism unleashed by an indexically more self-assured power,—biomedicine—ought to make this the right time for these systems to critically reevaluate their epistemic viability. And there is evidence that such a process is going on. And again it is hoped that this process will not end in unexamined capitulation to the technologically superior newcomer. There is a more important moral, if you will, to be learned from Siddha and similar traditional systems of healing and thought. Indexicality has not appropriated as much power to itself in Siddha medicine as it has in biomedicine. Some of this power, the power to persuade and to heal, is shared through iconicity, as has been demonstrated in our study of the pulse.

It is this prevailing presence of iconicity that has immunized Siddha medicine from such dichotomies as illness vs. disease and body vs. mind, and by extension, has made it epistemologically unnecessary if not impossible to invent such deprecatory labels such as "crocks," "gomers," "malingerers," and hypochondriacs (see George and Dundes 1978; Lipsitt 1970). In the absence of a mind-body dichotomy, phenomena such as "somatization" become meaningless and does not call for the kind of defence biomedical phychiatry finds necessary to construct (see Katon, Kleinman, and Rosen 1982).

Arguing against the unrelenting cartesianism in biomedicine, Hahn and Kleinman (1981) propose that we would serve the cause of health far more effectively if we conceived the body as mindful and the mind as embodied. In Siddha thought, such a conception is so fundamental that small pox is no more "real" than a "depressed heart," even though one may well be a more serious condition than the other. The bottom line in Siddha medicine is "suffering," as Hahn defines it in his paper in this volume. And given the significant part that iconicity plays in Siddha thought in general and in the diagnostic process in particular, suffering, any suffering, is not hermetically sealable by objectification, nor can non-suffering be masqueraded as suffering, an art for which epithets such as malingering and hypochondriasis have been reserved. Suffering is something that can be shared and must be shared by someone else, especially the physician.

In almost every one of the ethnographic essays in this volume the phenomenon of iconicity has been seen to operate. Most often this was expressed in terms of the transformation of a relationship of dis-ease that a person has with somebody or something into one of ease. In both Egnor's and Claus' essays dis-ease and suffering was dispelled when a disarticulated possession or oppression by a spirit of deity was changed into an articulated possession which brought about a certain measure of identity between subject and object. The avoidance of madness through the satiation of desire in Bhattacharyya's essay may also be seen as a merging through satiation of the desirer and the desired. The fulfilment of desire plays a similar role in Amarasingham's case study of the woman with a history of miscarriages. The dialogue between astrologer and client in Pugh's essay moves as much toward divining and advising as toward understanding, an understanding in which not only is an iconic relationship between the cognitive maps of astrologer and client sought but an iconicity into which planetary configurations enter as well.

The use of iconicity in healing is certainly not limited to Siddha, Ayurveda, or other homeopathic therapies. The phenomenon is a widespread one. A considerable portion of anthropological literature devoted to healing rituals have brought this to our attention, the best known among these being Victor Turner's (1968) study of Ndembu symbolism and Levi-Strauss' (1963) essay on "The Sorcerer and his Magic." The use of metaphor in psychotherapy is yet another example of iconicity at work in healing (see Erikson 1980; Bandler and Grinder 1979, 1981; Haley 1973). This turn of events in Western medical thought is encouraging. And for those who would rather relegate these attempts to a Tylorean vestige of sympathetic magic I would like to leave you, for whatever it is worth, the following event, recorded by a contemporary psychotherapist.

The case concerns a patient who had been catatonic for several years and abandoned to vegetate in a mental hospital in California. Bandler describes what happened:

"[He] had been sitting there for several years on the couch in the day room. The only communication he was offering me were his body position and his breathing rate. His eyes were open, pupils dilated. So I sat facing away from him at about a forty-five degree angle in a chair nearby, and I put myself in exactly the same body position, and I sat there for forty-five minutes breathing with him. At the end of forty minutes I had tried little variations in my breathing, and he would follow, so I knew I had rapport at that point. I could have changed my breathing slowly over a period of time and brought him out that way. Instead I interrupted and shocked him. I shouted, "Hey! Do you have a cigarette?" He jumped up off the coach and said "God! Don't do that!" (1979: 80).

NOTES

1   The greater part of the data on which this essay is based was obtained from Dr. R. Kannan of Tiruchirapalli, Tamil Nadu. Fiedlwork for this study was funded by the National Science Foundation which is acknowledged with gratitude.

2   Kandasamy Mudaliyar (1973: 48,49) ascribes these two quartrains to Tirumular's *Tirumandiram*. However, I have not been able to locate these among the 3,000 odd quartrains in the *Tirumandiram* and believe that they either belong to one of the minor poets of the eighteen *cittar* or has been passed down via an oral tradition that lies outside the published corpus of the eighteen *cittars'* compositions.

3   In keeping with the convention of citing from the *Collected Papers of C. S. Peirce*, the number to the left of the decimal point indicates the volume and that to the right indicates the paragraph.

4   That a patient is a sign may seem odd to those unfamiliar with Peirce's thought. For Peirce, man, is essentially a sign. For an explication of this perspective in the context of anthropological theory see Milton's Singer's essay, "Signs of the Self: An Exploration in Semiotic Anthropology" (1980)

5   This is quite clearly a hypothetical assumption, made for convenience rather than out of necessity. The physician may well be suffering from quite a different humoral imbalance. In either case the point holds: the physician's suffering-humor-pulse sign complex will not be the same as that of the patient. This is an important point to be taken note of. In Siddha medical theory no two persons, sick or otherwise, are constitutionally identical.

REFERENCES

BAER, Eugene
    1981   "Medical Semiotics: A New Paradigm," *Semiotica* 37(1/2): 165-191.
BANDLER, Richard, and John Grinder
    1979   *Frogs Into Princess: Neurolinguistic Programming*. Moab, Utah: Real People Press.
    1981   *Patterns of the Hypnotic Techniques of Milton H. Erikson*. 2. vols. Cupertino, California: Meta Publications.
DANIEL, E. Valentine
    1984   *Fluid Signs: Being a Person the Tamil Way*, Berkeley: University of California Press.
DEACON, Terrence W.
    1978   "Semiotics and Cybernetics: The Relevance of C. S. Peirce." In *Sanity and Signification*. Terrence W. Deacon, ed. Bellingham, Washington: Fairhaven College Publications.
ERIKSON, Milton H.
    1980   *The Collected Papers on Hypnosis*. 4 vols. Ernst L. Rossi, ed. New York: Irvington Publishers Inc.
FABREGA, Horacio, Jr., and Peter Manning
    1972   "Disease, Illness, and Deviant Careers." In *Theoretical Perspectives on Deviance*. R. A. Scott and J. D. Douglas, eds. New York: Basic Books.

FEINSTEIN, Alvin R.
1967 *Clinical Judgement*. Huntington, New York: Robert E. Krieger.
FITZGERALD, John J.
1966 *Peirce's Theory of Signs as Foundation for Pragmatism*. The Hague: Mouton and Company.
FOUCAULT, Michel
1965 *Madness and Civilization: A History of Insanity in the Age of Reason*. New York: Random House.
1973 *The Birth of the Clinic*. New York: Random House
1977 *Discipline and Punish. Birth of the Prison*. New York: Pantheon.
FOX, Renée C.
1980 "The Evolution of Medical Uncertainty." *Milbank Memorial Fund Quarterly* 58(1)
FRANKENBERG, Ronald
1980 "Medical Anthropology and Development: A Theoretical Perspective." *Social Science and Medicine* 14B: 197-207.
GEORGE, Victor and Allan DUNDES
'The Gomer. A Figure of American Hospital Folk Speech." Journal of American Folklore. 91(359): 568-581.
HAHN, Robert, and Arthur KLEINMAN
1981 "Belief as Pathogen, Belief as Medicine: 'Voodoo Death' and the 'Placebo Phenomenon' in Anthropological Perspective." Paper presented at the conference on "Symbols, Meaning, and Efficacy in the Healing Process," at Edinburgh Meeting of Society for Applied Anthropology.
HALEY, Jay.
1973 *Uncommon Therapy*. New York: W. W. Norton and Co.
KATON, Wayne, Arthur Kleinman, and Gary Rosen
1982 "Depression and Somatization. A Review. Parts I & II." *American Journal of Medicine*, 60(1 & 2).
KLEINMAN, Arthur, Leon EISENBERG, and Byron GOOD
1978 "Culture, Illness and Care." *Annals of Internal Medicine* 88(2): 251-258.
LEVI-STRAUSS, Claude
1967 *Structural Anthropology*. New York: Doubleday Anchor.
LIPSITT, Don R.
1970 "Medical and Psychological Characteristics of 'crocks.'" *Psychiatry in Medicine* 1(1).
MUDALIYAR, Kandasamy
1973 *Unavu Maruttuvam*. Madras: Metropolitan Press.
PEIRCE, Charles Sanders
1934 *Collected Papers*. Charles Hartshorne and Paul Weiss, eds. Cambridge: Harvard University Press.
PEIRCE, Charles Sanders and Victoria Lady WELBY
1977 *Semiotics and Significs. The Correspondence between Charles S. Peirce and Victoria Lady Welby*. Charles S. Hardwick, ed. Bloomington: Indiana University Press.
SILVERSTEIN, Michael
1976 "Shifters, Linguistic Categories and Cultural Description." In *Meaning in Anthropology*. Keith H. Basso and Henry Selby, eds. Alberquerque: University of New Mexico Press.
SINGER, Milton
1980 "Signs of the Self: An Exploration in Semiotic Anthropology." *American Anthropologist* 82(3): 485-507.
SONTAG, Susan
1977 *Illness as Metaphor*. New York: Random House.
SUDNOW, David
1979 *Passing On. The Social Organization of Dying*. Prentice Hall, Inc.: Englewood Cliffs, New Jersey.

Sydenham, Thomas
    1922 *Selected Works*. New York: W. Wood and Company.
Tirumular
    1972 *Tirumandiram* 2 Vols. P. Ramanatha Pillai, ed. Madras: Saiva Siddhanta Press.
Turner, Victor W.
    1967 *The Forest of Symbols*. Ithaca, New York: Cornell University Press.
Uexkull, Thure v., ed.
    1979 *Lehrbuch der Psychosomatischen Medizin*. Munchen: Urban und Schwarzberg.
Weiss, Paul, and Arthur Burks
    1945 "Peirce's Sixty Six signs." *Journal of Philosophy* 42: 383-388
Young, Allan
    1981 "The Anthropologies of Illness and Sickness. *Annual Review of Anthropology*. Palo Alto
           California: Annual Reviews
Zvelebil, Kamil
    1973 *The Smile of Murugan: On Tamil Literature in South India*. Leiden: E. J. Brill.
    1974 *Tamil Literature*. Wiesbaden: Otto Harrassowitz.

The Mādhavanidāna

and its chief commentary

Chapters 1-10

Introduction, translation and notes

by

G. J. MEULENBELD

(Orientalia Rheno-Traiectina, 19)

1974. (xii, 710 p.) (D)
ISBN 90 04 03892 2

cloth Gld. 168.—

The present work is a translation of the first ten chapters of Mādhava's Rogaviniścaya, usually referred to as the Mādhavanidāna, the earliest compendium of that section of traditional Indian medicine which is called nidāna and deals with aetiology, symptomatology and prognostics.

The translation of this text is presented together with an almost complete rendering of its chief commentary, the Madhukośa, and is accompanied by copious notes containing a.o. parallels from a series of important medical Sanskrit texts.

The volume also contains appendices treating the sources of the Mādhavanidām, the authors and works quoted, technical terms, Sanskrit names of plants and their botanical equivalents, and modern medical views on the diseases described in the text. It is concluded by a Sanskrit index, indices of botanical and zoological names, and a general index.

E. J. Brill — P.O.B. 9000 — 2300 PA Leiden — The Netherlands